PHYSICS FOR ANAESTHETISTS

PHYSICS FOR ANAESTHETISTS

By

JAMES DUFFIN, B.A.Sc., M.A.Sc., Ph.D.

Assistant Professor, Department of Anaesthesia
Assistant Professor, Department of Physiology
Member, Institute of Biomedical Engineering
University of Toronto
Toronto, Ontario, Canada

With a Foreword by

R. A. Gordon, C.D., M.D., F.R.C.P. (C), F.F.A.R.C.S. (Eng)

Professor and Chairman, Department of Anaesthesia
Faculty of Medicine, University of Toronto
Toronto, Ontario, Canada

CHARLES C THOMAS · PUBLISHER

Springfield · Illinois · U.S.A.

Published and Distributed Throughout the World by

CHARLES C THOMAS • PUBLISHER

Bannerstone House

301-327 East Lawrence Avenue, Springfield, Illinois, U.S.A

ISBN 0-398-03451-6

Library of Congress Catalog Card Number 75-12559

With THOMAS BOOKS careful attention is given to all details of manufacturing and design. It is the Publisher's desire to present books that are satisfactory as to their physical qualities and artistic possibilities and appropriate for their particular use. THOMAS BOOKS will be true to those laws of quality that assure a good name and good will.

Printed in the United States of America

C-1

Library of Congress Cataloging in Publication Data

Duffin, James.
Physics for anaesthetists.

Bibliography: p.
Includes index.
1. Anesthesiology—Apparatus and instruments.
I. Title. [DNLM: 1. Biophysics. 2. Physics.
3. Anesthesia. QT34 D757p]
RD82.D75 617'.96'0153 75-12559
ISBN 0-398-03451-6

FOREWORD

A BASIC KNOWLEDGE of physical science is fundamental to the understanding of biological phenomena, including the functions of the human body and aberrations of function due to disease, environment and the manipulations of the physician. Anaesthetists in particular also require a sound basic knowledge of physics for the intelligent application of the machinery which they use in patient care and monitoring systems.

While there is general agreement today that a knowledge of physics is essential to the anaesthetist, there still exist differences of opinion concerning the essential quantity and quality of that knowledge. There are undoubtedly those in the profession who believe that an ability to identify the gauges and to read and act upon the data displayed by the "black box" is more than adequate. However, if we are concerned with the application of science to improve the art of anaesthesia, then a more sophisticated knowledge of the derivation and meaning of pertinent physical phenomena is essential.

The preparation of a book designed to present the science of physics to clinicians is complicated by these disparate views of purpose. Undoubtedly in the recent past a text which relied extensively on mathematical statements would not have been understood by the majority of postgraduate students or practitioners in clinical disciplines. It is evident today, however, that the young physician achieves a much more sophisticated knowledge of mathematics than did his predecessors of a decade ago. It seems reasonable, then, in presenting physics to the anaesthetist, to take advantage of this educational advance. Dr. Duffin has done so in this volume, to great advantage. It is evident to this member of an earlier generation that the mathematical expressions can, in fact, be understood and that they are essential to the demonstration of the phenomena described. Moreover, the equations can all be solved easily with a modern pocket calculator.

Dr. Duffin's book will unquestionably be of tremendous value to postgraduate trainees in anesthesia, while a little effort expended in studying this text will undoubtedly make it possible for a much greater number of practitioners of the art to understand considerably more of the modern literature of the specialty.

R. A. GORDON

PREFACE

THE PRACTICE OF ANAESTHESIA is, in many respects, an art, but the determinants of such practice are based upon science. To understand and use the apparatus and techniques of anaesthesia, anaesthetists require a knowledge of basic physics. How much to acquire and to what depth are, as yet, unanswered questions.

This book emphasises fundamentals and a quantitative, analytical approach. The first, because while technology becomes obsolete, fundamental principles remain, and the second, because the nature of science is quantitative and analytical. It is my hope that anaesthetists, working through this book, will acquire not only an understanding of the basic physics which underlie anaesthetic practice, but also an analytical method in the application of such knowledge to the physical problems they encounter.

The writing of this book was not accomplished without help, and my gratitude extends to many people. I received expert advice on particular subjects from Mr. Russell G. K. Brown, Dr. David F. James, Dr. Charles A. Ward and Mr. Bruce R. Vachon. Dr. Ian C. G. Gallimore and Dr. Beverley A. Britt provided constructive criticism of the manuscript, as did many of the students in the postgraduate course in anaesthesia. I drew enthusiasm for this project from Dr. Charles H. Hockman and Dr. Edward Llewellyn-Thomas. Mrs. Marilyn Berg patiently and efficiently completed the complex typing of the manuscript. I am indebted to Dr. R. A. Gordon for the opportunity to pursue this endeavour, as well as for his continuing encouragement.

Toronto JAMES DUFFIN

ILLUSTRATIONS

TABLES

CONTENTS

PHYSICS FOR ANAESTHETISTS

Chapter 1

SYMBOLS AND FUNCTIONS

THE CONTENTS of this chapter constitute some elementary vocabulary and grammar in the language of mathematics. These form the basis of the following chapters as well as being directly applicable to some aspects of anaesthetic practice.

SYMBOLS

Before discussion can begin, it is necessary to translate some mathematical symbols into English. Table I lists commonly used mathematical symbols and their English translation. Some of these symbols are used without further explanation, while others are elaborated in the text as they are encountered. Table II lists the Greek alphabet, whose letters are often used in physics and engineering to denote specific quantities.

The reader is urged to view mathematical statements as a sort of shorthand method of writing a statement in English. For example, the mathematical statement,

$$C = \frac{V}{P},$$

TABLE I

MATHEMATICAL SYMBOLS

Symbol	Meaning	Symbol	Meaning
$+$	plus (addition)	$( ),\ < >,\ [\ ]$	parentheses
$-$	minus (subtraction)	$\rightarrow$	approaches
$\div,\ /$	division	ln	natural logarithm to the base e
$\times,\ \cdot$	multiplication (also xy denotes $x \cdot y$)	log	logarithm to the base 10
		∞	infinity
$=$	equal to	e	base of natural logarithms, 2.718 . . .
$\neq$	not equal to		
$\equiv$	equivalent to	Σ	the sum of
$>$	greater than	$\int$	the integral of
$<$	less than	$\frac{dy}{dx}$	the derivative of y with respect to x
$\simeq$	approximately equal to		
$\propto$	varies as	$\frac{dy}{dt},\ \dot{y}$	the derivative of y with respect to time, t.
$\surd$	square root		

TABLE II

GREEK ALPHABET (lower case)

α	alpha	ι	iota	ρ	rho
β	beta	κ	kappa	Σ σ	sigma
γ	gamma	λ	lambda	τ	tau
Δ δ	delta	μ	mu	υ	upsilon
ϵ	epsilon	ν	nu	ϕ	phi
ζ	zeta	ξ	xi	χ	chi
η	eta	o	omicron	ψ	psi
θ	theta	π	pi	ω	omega

should be read: C equals V divided by P. If we state that C denotes compliance, V, volume, and P, pressure, then the mathematical statement above says that compliance is equal to the ratio of volume divided by pressure.

The advantage of the mathematical statement lies not only in its brevity but also in its susceptibility to manipulation according to a set of mathematical rules. For example,

$$\frac{V}{P} = C.$$

Now, multiply both sides of the equation by P, thereby preserving the equality, to get

$$\frac{PV}{P} = PC,$$

and

$$V = PC.$$

In English, the statement above says that volume is equal to the product of pressure times compliance. This statement is not readily apparent from the original statement in English but is easily derived from the original mathematical statement.

In addition to the translation of mathematical symbols before discussion starts, it is also necessary to define the terms constant, parameter and variable. A *constant* is rigorously defined as a quantity which maintains a fixed value for all situations and all time. Constants are usually symbolized by capital letters of the alphabet in mathematical statements while well-known constants such as π (3.1416) use letters of the Greek alphabet.

Often, constants are arbitrary in the sense that the quantity only maintains a fixed value for specific situations and periods of time. Such quantities are called *parameters* and are usually symbolized by capital letters of the alphabet. For example, C, symbolizing the compliance of the lungs, is often assumed to be constant in any particular patient for a period of time but actually changes from patient to patient and from time to time.

A *variable* is a quantity which has a changing value throughout the course of a situation. Variables are often symbolized by lower case letters from the end of the alphabet, for example, x, y and z.

STRAIGHT LINES

Anaesthetists, like most people, have a tendency to think of the relationships between causes and effects as being proportional. During artificial ventilation, for example, it may be observed that the greater the mouth pressure is, the larger the expanded volume of the lungs. Measured values of the increase in lung volume, resulting from different mouth pressures, may be plotted on a graph of volume increase against pressure such as that

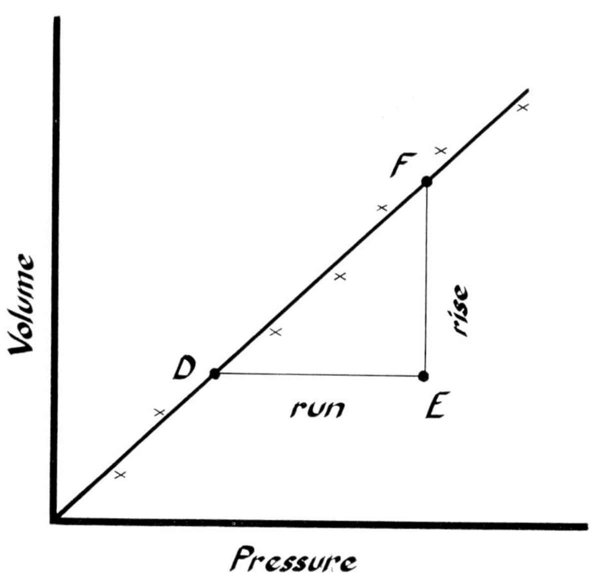

Figure 1. Slope of a straight line.

of Figure 1. If the plotted experimental points can be joined by a straight line, then there is said to be a linear relationship between volume and pressure.

The characteristic which distinguishes this particular line from others is its inclination with respect to the axes of the graph (the axes are volume and pressure). The inclination is measured by a quantity termed the *slope* of the line. In Figure 1, start at point D on the line and *run* horizontally to point E. Then, *rise* vertically back to the line at point F. The slope of the line is defined as the rise divided by the run.

$$slope = \frac{rise}{run} = \frac{\mathrm{EF}}{\mathrm{DE}}$$

The slope of a line may be positive, as in Figure 1, or negative. For a line sloping downwards to the right the rise would be negative, i.e. a fall; the slope of the line would therefore be negative.

The slope of the line shown in Figure 1 is the amount by which volume increases for any particular increase in pressure, divided by that pressure increase. We can recognize the slope as total compliance, the constant of proportionality between volume and pressure. Symbolically,

$$V \propto P$$

and

$$V = CP$$

so,

$$C = \frac{V}{P} = slope,$$

where V, C, and P are symbols standing for volume increase, compliance and mouth pressure respectively. C is a parameter, constant for this particular set of measurements, while V and P are variables. In keeping with the cause and effect reasoning, V is called the *dependent variable* because its value is determined by the value of P. P is therefore termed the *independent variable*, determined by the anaesthetist controlling the ventilator. By convention, the dependent variable is usually written on the left-hand side of the equation.

In generalized mathematical statements, y is usually the dependent variable and either x or time, t, the independent variable. One useful form of the generalized equation for a straight line is

$$y = mx + b$$

where:

x is the independent variable,
y is the dependent variable,
m is a parameter, the slope of the line,
b is a parameter, the y-intercept.

The equation above is plotted on a graph in Figure 2. The slope of the line is m, and the line intersects the y-axis at a value of b, called the y-intercept. Particular values of m and b represent specific lines. For example:

$m \to \infty$ is a vertical line, the y-axis,
$m = 0$ is a horizontal line, b units away from the x-axis,
$b = 0$ is a line through the origin (the origin is the point of intersection of the x and y axes).

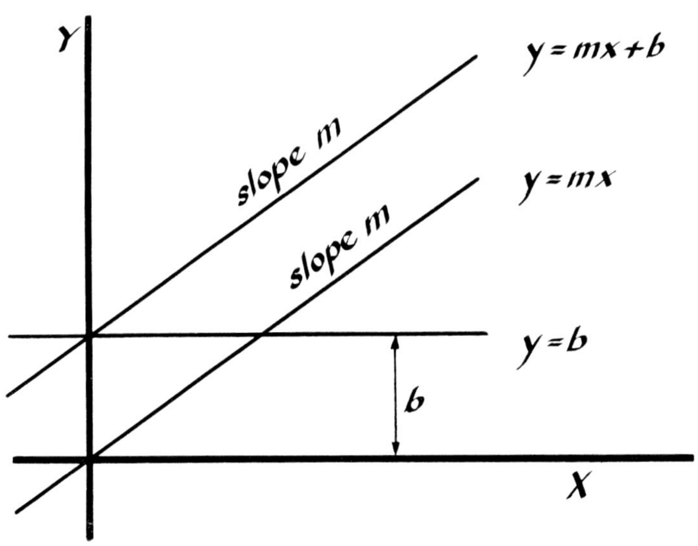

Figure 2. General form of the straight line.

CURVES

In many cases, the relationship between two quantities may not be a simple proportion, but may form a curve when plotted on a graph. In this case, there are many other equations which may fit the plotted data. Consider the equation

$$y = x^2$$

(Recall that x^2 means $x \cdot x$.) To plot this equation on a rectangular coordinate system as shown in Figure 3, make a table of values for x and y by assuming values for x, the independent variable, and calculating y from the equation.

The curve shown in Figure 3 is called a *parabola*. Unlike the

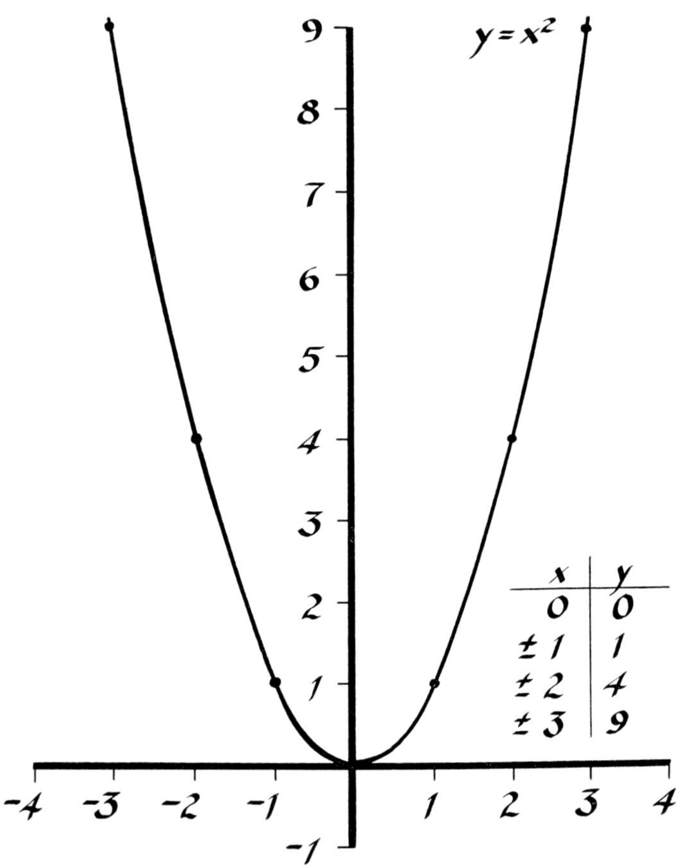

Figure 3. Plot of the equation, $y = x^2$.

straight line, the slope of the parabola changes with different values of the independent variable x. In fact, the slope at any point on the curve is different from that at any other point. The determination of the slope at any particular point on the curve is discussed in Chapter 2.

There are many equations available to describe the curves assumed by graphical data, some simple as in the example above, and others more complex:

$$y = Ax^3 + Bx^2 + Cx + D$$

where x and y are the independent and dependent variables respectively, and A, B, C and D are parameters.

In general, the expression on the right-hand side of the equation involving x is called a *function* of x. The dependency of one variable, y, upon another, x, is often expressed by stating that y is a function of x, without actually specifying a particular function. The dependency is expressed symbolically as,

$$y = f(x).$$

The function of x, $f(x)$, might be complex such as the previous example, or a simple linear function like the straight line equation discussed earlier, or it could be trigonometric.

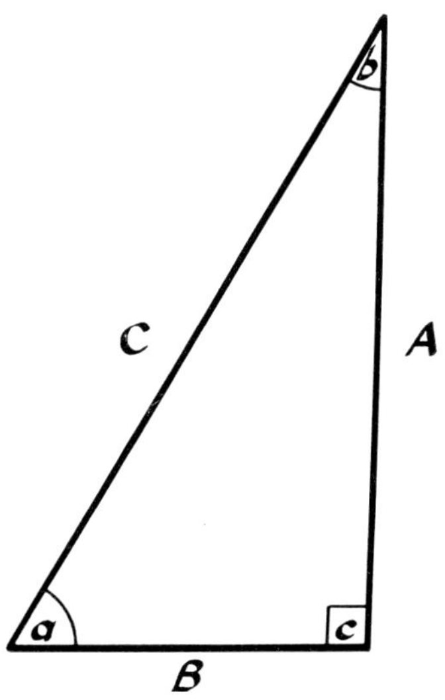

Figure 4. Right-angled triangle.

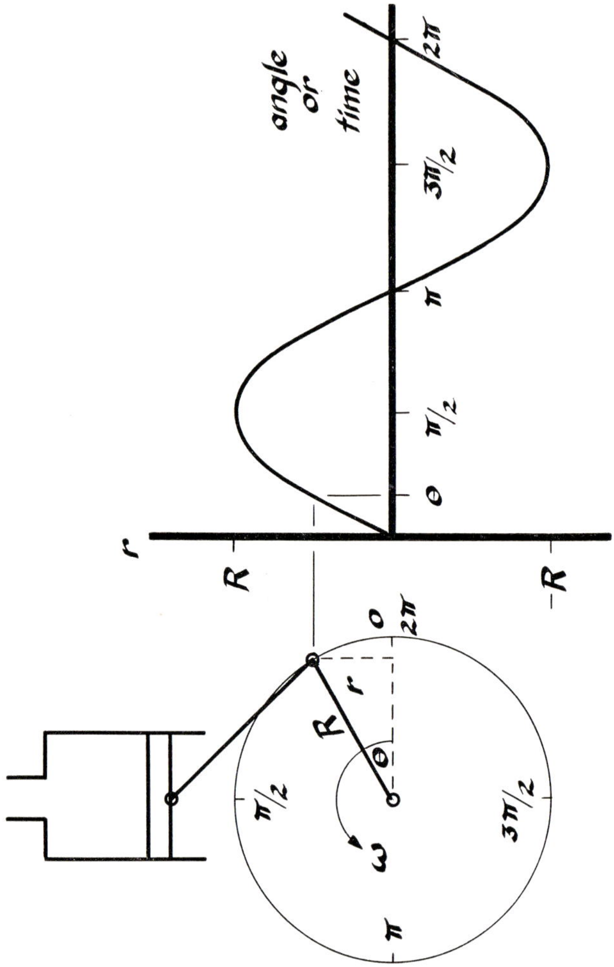

Figure 6. Generation of a sine wave.

Figure 6 shows the generation of a sine wave motion of a piston driven by a rotating crank. The assertion that the position of the piston varies as a sine function of time may be proven as follows.

First, define the symbols for the constants and variables of the mechanical system:

r = the distance from the crank pin to a horizontal line running through the axle, at any time t.

t = the time elapsed since the crank left the horizontal starting position (in seconds).

θ = the angle (theta) in radians between the crank position at any time, t, and the crank position at the start.

ω = the constant angular speed of rotation (omega) of the crank in radians/second.

R = the constant length of the crank.

Now we may state the relationships between these quantities by examining Figure 6. The crank traverses an angle, θ, at a speed of ω; so,

$$\theta = \omega t.$$

Angle θ is also related to the variable, r, and constant, R, trigonometrically since a right angle triangle is formed by sides r, R and the horizontal line through the axle. From the definition of $\sin\theta$,

$$\sin\theta = \frac{r}{R}$$

and

$$r = R\sin\theta.$$

Substituting, $\theta = \omega t$ into the equation above yields

$$r = R\sin\omega t.$$

We can plot a graph of the variation of r with respect to either t or θ as shown in Figure 6. The variation of r with time repeats at each revolution of the wheel and is called a sine wave. The *amplitude* of the sine wave is the length of the crank arm R, and the time taken for one revolution is called the *period* T. Its reciprocal, the number of revolutions, or cycles, per second is called the *frequency*, f, of the sine wave. Stated symbolically,

$$1 \text{ revolution or cycle} = 2\pi \text{ radians;}$$

therefore,

$$\text{time taken for 1 cycle} = \frac{\theta}{\omega} = \frac{2\pi}{\omega}$$

and

$$T = \frac{2\pi}{\omega} \text{ seconds;}$$

so,

$$f = \frac{1}{T} = \frac{\omega}{2\pi} \left(\frac{1}{\text{seconds}} \text{ or } \text{seconds}^{-1}\right) \text{Hz.}$$

The unit of frequency, seconds^{-1}, has been named the hertz, in honour of Heinrich Rudolf Hertz (1857-1894), the German physicist, and is abbreviated Hz, in the S.I. units to be detailed in Chapter 4.

Having described the motion of the crank pin as a sine wave, it can be seen that the piston, directly attached to the crank pin, will move up and down with a sine wave motion, causing air flow in and out of the cylinder which may also vary sinusoidally. Several ventilators are operated on this principle (for example the Starling pump, the Engström ventilator and the electrically operated Emerson ventilator), and produce lung inflations with sinusoidal characteristics, although they may be distorted by compliance effects and cycling mechanisms.

LOGARITHMS AND EXPONENTIALS

The logarithmic and exponential functions are interrelated and of particular use to anaesthetists. Consider that the large number, one hundred thousand may be written more easily in exponential form as

$$100000 = 10^5.$$

The 5 is referred to as the index or exponent, and it signifies that five tens are to be multipled together to get one hundred thousand. The 5 may also be referred to as the logarithm of one hundred thousand to the base ten. The same statement as above written in logarithmic form is thus,

$$\log_{10}(100000) = 5,$$

so the logarithmic notation is a second method of expressing exponential relationships.

The logarithm, or exponential, method of expressing very large or very small numbers is extremely useful. Rather than state a hydrogen ion concentration in moles per litre as, 0.0000001 or 1/10000000, we may say it is 10^{-7}. (The negative exponent signifies that the reciprocal of seven tens are to be multiplied together to get one ten-millionth.) With frequent usage, we define pH as the negative logarithm (to the base ten) of the hydrogen ion concentration in moles per litre and say pH = 7.

In general terms, the logarithm, *L*, of a number, *N*, to a given base, *B*, is the exponent of the base which gives the number. In symbols,

$$L = \log_B (N)$$

is another way of writing

$$B^L = N.$$

Because logarithms are exponents they have useful properties; for example, two numbers may be multiplied together by adding their respective logarithms to obtain the logarithm of the product. In this way, a difficult multiplication may be changed to a simple addition. Tables are available for logarithms of numbers so as to make it easy to find the logarithm of any number, and tables listing the number for any given logarithm, called antilog tables, make it easy to determine the answer to the problem having found the logarithm of the answer. The slide rule is analogous to tables of logarithms. The useful properties of logarithms are listed below:

$$\log (MN) = \log(M) + \log(N)$$

$$\log \left(\frac{M}{N}\right) = \log(M) - (N)$$

$$\log (M^n) = n\log(M)$$

$$\log (\sqrt[n]{M}) = \log (M^{1/n}) = \frac{1}{n} \log(M)$$

In exponential form these properties appear as follows:

$$B^m \cdot B^n = B^{m+n}$$

$$\frac{B^m}{B^n} = B^{m-n}$$

$$(B^m)^n = B^{m \cdot n}$$

$$\sqrt[n]{B^m} = (B^m)^{1/n} = B^{m/n}$$

Logarithms to the base of 10 are called common or *Briggsian logarithms* after Henry Briggs (1561-1630), the English mathematician who invented them. When the base is unspecified it is usually taken as 10. Other bases may be used such as 2 (for the binary numbers in computers), and the irrational number $e = 2.718\ldots$. Logarithms to the base e are called natural or *Napierian logarithms* after their inventor John Napier (1550-1617), a Scottish mathematician, and abbreviated ln; for example,

$$\ln(N) = L,$$

is another way of writing,

$$e^L = N.$$

The conversion factors between common and natural logarithms are:

$$\ln(N) = 2.303 \quad \log(N),$$

$$\log(N) = 0.4343 \ln(N).$$

The logarithmic function can be plotted on a graph using the equation below which states that the dependent variable, y, is a logarithmic function of the independent variable, x.

$$y = \log_2(x).$$

Figure 7 shows y plotted against x. Note that when $x = 1$, $y = 0$. The graph may have a familiar shape because it shows the Weber-Fechner generalization, that the output, y, of a biological receptor system, such as touch, hearing and sight, varies as a logarithmic function of the stimulus, x. The Weber-Fechner law was named after its discoverer Ernst Heinrich Weber (1795-1878), the German physiologist, and its popularizer Gustav Theodor Fechner (1801-1887), the German physicist and philosopher.

Similarly, the exponential function may be graphed by consid-

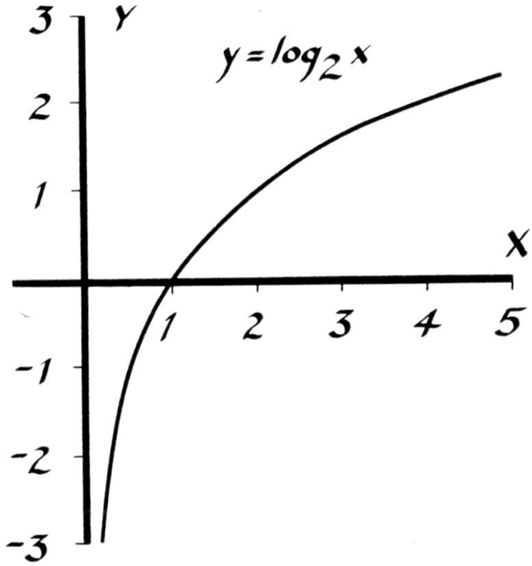

Figure 7. Plot of the logarithmic function.

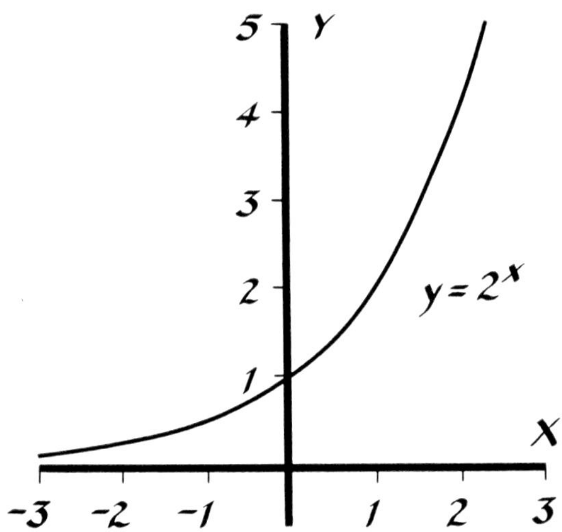

Figure 8. Plot of the exponential function.

ering y, the dependent variable, as an exponential function of x, the independent variable. The base 2 was chosen; so,

$$y = 2^x.$$

Figure 8 shows y as an exponential function of x, a curve the same as the logarithmic function but reoriented with respect to the x and y axes. Note that when $x = 0$, $y = 1$ because

$$y = 2^0 = 2^{1-1} = 2/2 = 1.$$

The graph shows that as x increases positively, y increases at an ever increasing rate so that this portion of the graph describes a run-away system such as unchecked bacterial growth, where y represents the total population and x represents time or the number of generations. The graph also shows that as x becomes more and more negative, y approaches zero. This portion of the graph is called a negative exponential curve and will be discussed at length in Chapter 3 as it is of considerable importance to anaesthetists.

PROBLEM 1

a) Plot the relationship,

$$y = \frac{1}{x}$$

on rectangular coordinates, and name the curve produced. This curve describes the relation between the pressure and volume of an ideal gas at a constant temperature.

b) The volume, in litres, inside the cylinder of a sine wave ventilator varies according to the equation,

$$V = 0.25 \sin(0.6\ \pi t)$$

What is the stroke volume in millilitres, and the frequency in Hz and breaths/minute for this ventilator?

Chapter 2

ELEMENTARY CALCULUS

DIFFERENTIATION

IN THE FIRST CHAPTER, the slope of a straight line was defined as rise/run and was observed to be the same no matter what part of the straight line was examined. However, the slope of a curve, like the parabola, $y = x^2$, shown in Figure 9, was observed to vary from point to point on the curve.

If we choose a point, P, on the parabola where $x = 2$ and try to

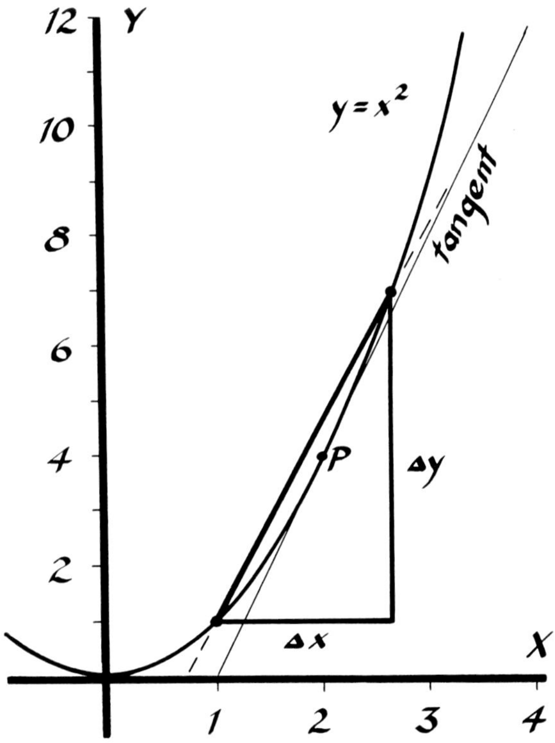

Figure 9. Slope of a curve.

find the slope by dividing Δy by Δx, we will only estimate the slope. The thin solid line is the *tangent* to the curve at point P, a line running through P with its slope equal to that of the curve at point P. Compare the slope of the estimate, dashed line, with that of the tangent. A more accurate estimate could be made if the run was smaller; that is, Δx reduced in size, but the slope of the parabola at point P would still not be determined exactly. In order to achieve an exact measurement of the slope, Δx would have to be reduced to the smallest possible length, i.e. zero. The value of the slope, $\Delta y/\Delta x$, when $\Delta x \rightarrow 0$, is called the *derivative* of y with respect to x and written:

$$\frac{dy}{dx} = \underset{\Delta x \rightarrow 0}{\text{limit of}} \left(\frac{\Delta y}{\Delta x}\right)$$

The mathematical process of finding the limiting value of $\Delta y/\Delta x$ as Δx approaches zero is called *differentiation*, and the result, dy/dx, is the slope of the parabola at point P where $x = 2$. dy and dx are called differentials, minute changes in the values of y and x, virtually equal to zero. Because the process of differentiation is a tedious mathematical procedure, formulas have been prepared which give the derivative for commonly used functions. The formula that we need in order to find the slope of the parabola at point P is as follows:
for $y = Kx^n$;

$$\frac{dy}{dx} = Knx^{n-1}$$

where n is equal to any integer and K is a constant.

For the parabola $y = x^2$; $n = 2$ and $K = 1$ so

$$\frac{dy}{dx} = 2x^{2-1} = 2x.$$

The statement above says that the slope (dy/dx) of the parabola ($y = x^2$) at any point on the curve is equal to $2x$. In other words the slope is a function of x. Since point P lies at $x = 2$, then the slope of the parabola there is $2 \times 2 = 4$. A straight line drawn through point P with this slope is called the tangent to the curve at point P.

The differentiation formulas for two other functions will be useful later.
For $y = K$;

$$\frac{dy}{dx} = 0,$$

and for $y = Kz$;

$$\frac{dy}{dx} = K\frac{dz}{dx},$$

where: K is a constant, and x, y and z are variables.

The first formula states that the derivative of a constant is equal to zero. Geometrically, $y = K$ would plot on $x - y$ coordinates as a horizontal line K units away from the x-axis. The slope of a horizontal line is zero so $dy/dx = 0$ for $y = K$. Logically, if $y = K$, a constant, then K doesn't change with respect to x. dy/dx (slope) measures the change of y resulting from a change in x; so in this case it is zero.

The second formula states that the derivative of a constant times a variable is equal to the product of the constant times the derivative of the variable.

One further rule of differentiation should be stated. It is that the derivative of a sum or difference is equal to the sum or difference of the derivatives. Symbolically,

$$\frac{d}{dx}(y \pm z) = \frac{dy}{dx} \pm \frac{dz}{dx},$$

How does the mathematical concept of differentiation apply to the real world? The most common example of a derivative is the rate of change of a quantity with time, for instance the spirometer tracings shown in Figure 10. Tracing A rises linearly with time, the inspiration generated by a constant flow ventilator. The rate of change of volume with time is flow and is the slope of the straight line A. In this case flow is determined easily by measuring the slope of the line, without recourse to differentiation formulas. However, consider tracing B, the spirometer trace of an actual inspiration. In this case flow, the slope of the line, changes from moment to moment. We can only specify flow at a given time as the derivative of volume with respect to time.

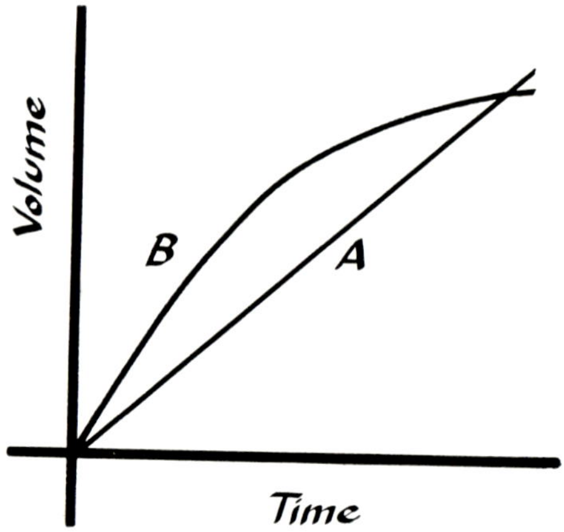

Figure 10. Examples of spirometer traces.

Differentiation is necessary here because flow itself, as well as volume, is changing with time.

Flow may be defined, in terms of volume, as the rate of change of volume with respect to time, or the slope of the volume versus time graph, or the derivative of volume with respect to time. The commonly used definition of flow as a given volume per unit time is only true if flow is constant. If flow is changing with time it must be expressed either as instantaneous flow, the derivative of volume with respect to time, or as an average flow over a set period of time.

INTEGRATION

Continuing the breathing example, we could have measured the flow of air with a pneumotachograph to obtain the rate of change (derivative) of volume with respect to time directly. Now suppose that we wish to find volume, having been given its derivative (flow). The process may be thought of as a sort of reverse differentiation and is called *integration.* Suppose the graph of flow against time was very simply that shown in Figure 11, where flow is constant at a value of 100 ml/second.

If we wished to determine the volume accumulated in the first three seconds of time, we would simply multiply flow times time,

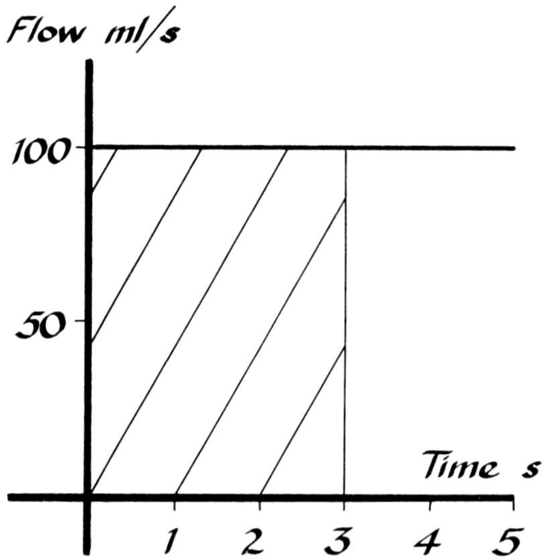

Figure 11. Area beneath a straight line.

i.e. 3 seconds × 100 ml/second, to get 300 ml. Now, note that flow × time is the area of the shaded rectangle of length 3 seconds and width 100 ml/second; in other words, the volume accumulated in three seconds is the area under the flow trace.

From this simple example we can see that given flow, the derivative of volume with respect to time, we can find the accumulated volume in a sort of reverse differentiation by geometrically determining the area beneath the flow versus time graph. This procedure is an elementary form of integration. However, consider the graph of flow, F, against time, t, shown in Figure 12. It is a parabolic curve described by the equation,

$$F = 10t^2,$$

where: F = flow in ml/second,
t = time in seconds.

The volume accumulated during the first three seconds of flow is the area beneath the parabolic curve. We could calculate the area by dividing it into triangles and rectangles as shown in Figure 12, but the areas are not quite triangular due to the curva-

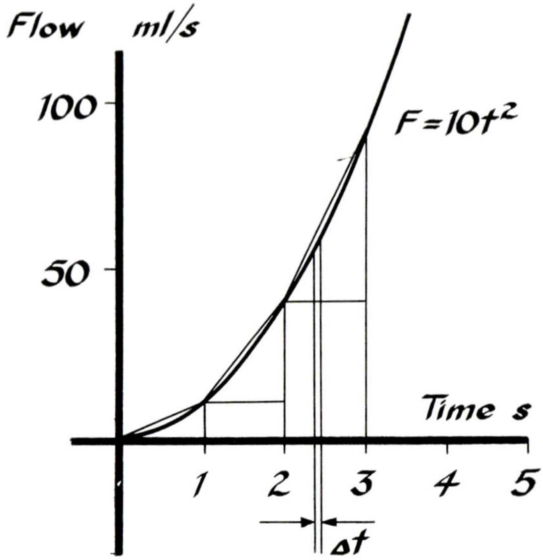

Figure 12. Area beneath a curve.

ture of the parabola, and so only an approximation is obtained. A better estimate could be made if we used smaller time intervals, dividing the area beneath the flow curve into slices Δt thick. The total area would then be approximated by the sum of the areas of the rectangles; Δt times the average flow during that small interval of time. We could write such a summation symbolically as,

$$V = \sum_{t=0}^{t=3} (\overline{F} \cdot \Delta t),$$

where: V = volume,

$\overline{F}$ = average flow during time Δt

Δt = a small period of time,

$\sum_{t=0}^{t=3}$ means the sum of the bracketed products from $t = 0$ to $t = 3$.

The volume found by this method is still not exact however, and what must be done is to reduce the thickness of the slices (Δt) to zero, and then add up all the areas of the slices. This may be done mathematically by the process called integration, written symbolically as,

$$V = {}_0\int^3 F \cdot dt.$$

The statement above should be read as: Volume equals the definite integral of flow with respect to time, from $t = 0$ to $t = 3$. The operation is known as integration between limits, $t = 0$ being the lower limit and $t = 3$ the upper limit. If the limits are omitted, the integral is indefinite, and a constant of integration must be added.

As in the case of differentiation, there are formulas for integration too, and the one that we require for our problem is, for $y = Kx^n$;

$$_0\int^x y \cdot dx = \frac{Kx^{n+1}}{n+1}$$

where: y is the dependent variable,
x is the independent variable,
K is a constant,
n is the exponent, any integer except, -1.

Using this formula we may determine the volume moved in the first three seconds of the parabolic flow versus time relation of Figure 12 as follows:

$$F = 10t^2;\ V = {}_0\int^3 F \cdot dt = \frac{10\ t^{2+1}}{2+1}$$

and,

$$V = \frac{10t^3}{3}$$

The area from $t = 0$ to $t = 3$ is found by putting $t = 3$ in the result of integration,

$$V = \frac{10t^3}{3} \text{ for } t = 3 \text{ is } \frac{10 \times 27}{3} = 90 \text{ ml.}$$

So the area beneath the flow curve, that is the volume accumulated from $t = 0$ to $t = 3$, is 90 ml. If we wished to obtain the volume accumulated between the second and third seconds, then we would have to subtract the volume accumulated between $t = 0$ and $t = 2$ from the volume accumulated between $t = 0$ and $t = 3$. The integration process would then be written symbolically as follows:

$$V = {}_2\int^3 F \cdot dt = {}_2\int^3 10t^2dt$$

$$V = \left[\frac{10t^3}{3}\right]_{t=2}^{t=3}$$

$$V = \left(\frac{270}{3}\right) - \left(\frac{80}{3}\right)$$

$$V = \frac{190}{3} = 63.3 \text{ ml.}$$

These two examples have shown that integration may be viewed as the reverse of differentiation. Because we may say that flow is the derivative of volume with respect to time, we may also state that volume is the integral of flow with respect to time. Volume may be defined, in terms of flow, as the accumulation of flow with time, or the area beneath the flow versus time graph, or the integral of flow with respect to time. The commonly used method of obtaining volume from flow by multiplying flow times time is only true if flow is constant. If flow is changing with time, then the volume accumulating must be expressed as the integral of flow with respect to time.

Two other formulas for integration which will be useful in later discussions are:

for $y = \frac{K}{x} = Kx^{-1}$;

$$\int y \cdot dx = K \cdot \ln x + C,$$

and for $y = K$;

$$\int y \cdot dx = Kx + C,$$

where: y is the dependent variable,
x is the independent variable,
K is a constant,
C is the constant of integration.

The first integration formula is extremely useful in the biological sciences and will be used later in an application to anaesthetics. The second formula merely states formally that the integration of a constant with respect to an independent variable is simply the product of the two, as we had already discovered in the constant flow example.

These formulas for integration are written for the indefinite integral, rather than the definite integral used in the example, and therefore include a constant of integration, C. The constant is the value of the integral up until the time, unspecified or indefinite, that is eventually chosen to start the integration. In the last example, we decided to begin integration at $t = 2$. The total integral, however, includes the volume from $t = 0$ to $t = 2$, and so we would add 80/3 ml as a constant of integration for this choice of starting time.

So far both integration and differentiation have been carried out by geometric approximations and by the exact calculus. The latter technique may only be used when the graph is a known mathematical function, and both methods may only be used in retrospect. Another approach is to employ machines (called respectively an *integrator* and *differentiator*) to calculate the integral or derivative with respect to time as the event of interest takes place, i.e. in real time.

Perhaps the most common examples of integrators used in anesthesia are the electronic integrator, used to obtain volume measurements by integrating the flow signal from a pneumotachograph, and the Wright Respirometer which mechanically integrates flow to obtain volume. The concept of the integration constant is more easily understood in the case of integrators as the amount already accumulated by the integrator before the period of interest to the observer. The differentiator is also used. Currently, the maximum rate of change of left ventricular pressure is used as an index of myocardial contractility, and this measurement may be obtained by using a differentiator to differentiate the pressure with respect to time.

Integrators and differentiators include many mechanical devices, analogue computer circuits, and digital computer programs. These machines perform the tedious calculations in real time, as the changes occur, rather than in retrospect as we did in the examples.

DIFFERENTIAL EQUATIONS

In an anaesthetized patient, during passive expiration the maximum expiratory flow depends upon the lung volume attained during the previous inspiration. In a single expiration the flow is high initially and declines as the volume of the lungs declines. We know or can intuitively guess that the higher the lung volume during a single passive expiration, the proportionately faster the air leaves, because we have all noticed that water leaks from a vessel more rapidly when it is full than when it is half empty. Here is another example of our tendency to seek for linear relationships between cause and effect. Assume that the air flow, F, during passive expiration is proportional to the volume, V, that is left to empty;

$$F \propto V$$

and if the proportionality constant is K then

$$F = K \cdot V,$$

a linear equation. The outflow, F, is, in fact, the rate of decline of lung volume, V, with respect to time, t. That is to say,

$$F = -\frac{dV}{dt},$$

the negative sign indicating a fall in volume. The equation describing the passive expiration is thus,

$$F = \frac{-dV}{dt} = K \cdot V.$$

The equation is a straight line passing through the origin with slope K, as shown in Figure 13. It is called a differential equation because it contains the differentials dV and dt.

Differential equations are solved by integrating both sides and thereby eliminating the differentials. The integration may be done by a machine, such as solution by simulation of the equation on an analog computer where an electrical analogue is set up to mimic the actual emptying of the lungs, or the integration may be done by calculus using a classical approach. The latter will be used here. The classical approach consists of manipulat-

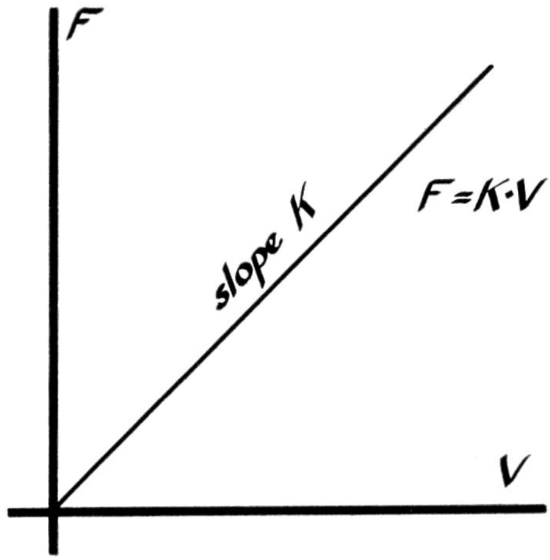

Figure 13. Plot of outflow versus volume remaining, for a hypothetical, passive expiration.

ing both sides of the equation until they conform to functions for which there are integration formulas.

We may solve our differential equation (manipulating it into a form that can be integrated so as to eliminate the differentials) by crossmultiplying, that is multiplying both sides by $-dt/V$ to get,

$$\left(\frac{-dV}{dt}\right)\left(\frac{-dt}{V}\right) = K \cdot V\left(\frac{-dt}{V}\right),$$

and

$$\frac{dV}{V} = -K \cdot dt.$$

Now, recall the last two integration formulas:

$$\int \frac{dx}{x} = \ln x + C_1$$

and

$$\int Kdx = Kx + C_2$$

where C_1 and C_2 are the integration constants.

Now integrate both sides of the differential equation, that is,

$$\int \frac{dV}{V} = \int -Kdt,$$

becomes

$$\ln V + C_1 = -K \cdot t + C_2$$

Subtract C_1 from both sides to get,

$$\ln V = -K \cdot t + (C_2 - C_1).$$

Consider the definition of natural logarithms. If the natural logarithm of V is $-K \cdot t + (C_2 - C_1)$, then $-K \cdot t + (C_2 - C_1)$ is the exponent of e which gives V, so,

$$V = e^{(-K \cdot t + C_2 - C_1)},$$

and since the exponents of products with the same base add, then

$$V = e^{-Kt} \cdot e^{(C_2 - C_1)}.$$

The constant $e^{(C_2 - C_1)}$, may be found from the boundary or starting condition that at the beginning of expiration when $t = 0$, then $V = V_T$, the tidal volume. Substitute these known values of time and volume into the equation and solve for $e^{(C_2 - C_1)}$ as follows:

$$V_T = e^{-K \cdot 0} \cdot e^{(C_2 - C_1)},$$
$$V_T = e^{0} \cdot e^{(C_2 - C_1)},$$

Since

$$e^{0} = e^{1-1}\ e/e = 1,$$

therefore,

$$V_T = e^{(C_2 - C_1)},$$

and the constant $e^{(C_2 - C_1)}$ is equal to V_T, the lung volume at the beginning of expiration. The final version of the expiration equation is

$$V = V_T\ e^{-K \cdot t},$$

and Figure 14 shows lung volume, V, versus time, t, during a passive expiration. Lung volume starts at a value V_T and falls along a negative exponential curve to zero as time goes on.

This example solution of a simple differential equation was included here, not because anaesthetists need to be mathematicians, but because the solution is a typical one. The principle that a dependent variable (lung volume in the example) decreases with time (the independent variable) at a rate proportional to the amount of the dependent variable still remaining is widespread in biology. Since rate of decrease with time is sy-

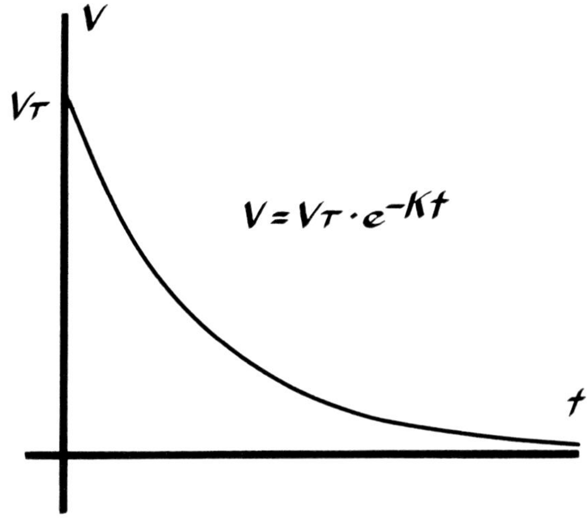

Figure 14. Plot of volume remaining versus time, for a hypothetical, passive expiration.

nonymous with negative derivative with respect to time, the principle implies a differential equation; the negative derivative of the dependent variable with respect to time is proportional to the dependent variable itself. The method of solution is always similar to our example, and the result, the variation of the dependent variable with time, is always some form of negative exponential curve. Therefore, aware of the method of solution, we know that a negative exponential variation with time, or a differential equation made up of a negative derivative of a variable, proportional to the variable, or the principle of decrease at a rate proportional to the amount left, all imply each other.

PROBLEM 2

Given that:

$$y = 3x^3,$$

find (a) the slope of the curve for $x = 2$ and (b) the area under the curve from $x = 2$ to $x = 4$.

Chapter 3

THE NEGATIVE EXPONENTIAL FUNCTION

PROPERTIES

THE NEGATIVE EXPONENTIAL function, or exponential decay curve, is of fundamental importance to the anaesthetist. Examples of it are passive expiration, the elimination of anaesthetics and other drugs, the changes in arterial P_{CO_2} and P_{O_2} after step changes in ventilation, and the downslope of dye dilution curves.

The negative exponential function results from the law of decrease by constant proportion; the quantity under consideration decreases at a rate proportional to the amount still present. Consider the example of passive expiration discussed in the last chapter. Figure 13 showed the law of decrease by constant proportion for V, the lung volume, stated as,

$$\text{expiratory flow} = -\frac{dV}{dt} = K \cdot V,$$

and Figure 14 showed the variation of volume with time which resulted, stated as,

$$V = V_T \cdot e^{-K \cdot t}$$

Now, consider the above equation as plotted in Figure 15. At any point P on the curve, we can draw a tangent to the curve, that is a straight line passing through point P with a slope equal to that of the curve at point P. The slope of the curve at point P is dV/dt, and we already know that $dV/dt = -K \cdot V$ from the law of decrease by constant proportion that we started with; so the slope at point P is $-K \cdot V_1$.

In Figure 15, the tangent is drawn in, together with a perpendicular line through P to the time axis. The sides of the triangle

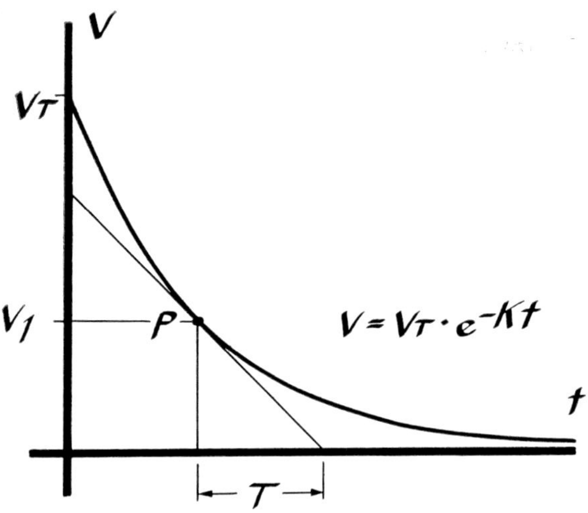

Figure 15. Time constant of a negative exponential curve.

formed by the perpendicular, the tangent and the time axis can be related to the slope of the tangent as follows:

$$\text{tangent slope} = \frac{rise}{run} = -\frac{V_1}{run} = -K \cdot V_1$$

The unknown quantity in this equation is the *run*, the distance along the time axis between the perpendicular and the tangent. From the above equation,

$$run = \frac{-V_1}{-K \cdot V_1} = \frac{1}{K}.$$

The quantity, $1/K$, is a length of the time axis, so it is measured in units of time and is called the *time constant*, T, defined as,

$$T = \frac{1}{K}$$

The time constant completely characterizes the shape of the negative exponential curve because it is the inverse of the proportionality constant which determines the function. The geometric construction shown in Figure 15 may be made at any point on the negative exponential curve, and the distance along the time axis between the tangent and the perpendicular will always be equal to T, the time constant.

We may also note that when time, t, in the negative exponential equation,

$$V = V_T \cdot e^{-t/T},$$

becomes equal to T then,

$$V = V_T \cdot e^{-T/T},$$

$$V = V_T \cdot e^{-1},$$

$$V = \frac{V_T}{e},$$

so that T may also be defined as the time required for volume to decay to a value $1/e$ times the starting value. Note too that the starting time may be any choice and the argument above still applies, that T units further on in time the value of V at the chosen starting time will have decayed to V/e.

To explain the property of the curve in another way, we could say that one part of the negative exponential curve differs from another part only by a scale factor. To illustrate what is meant by this statement Figure 16 shows y declining exponentially with time, t, at a time constant of T. When y declines to half its initial

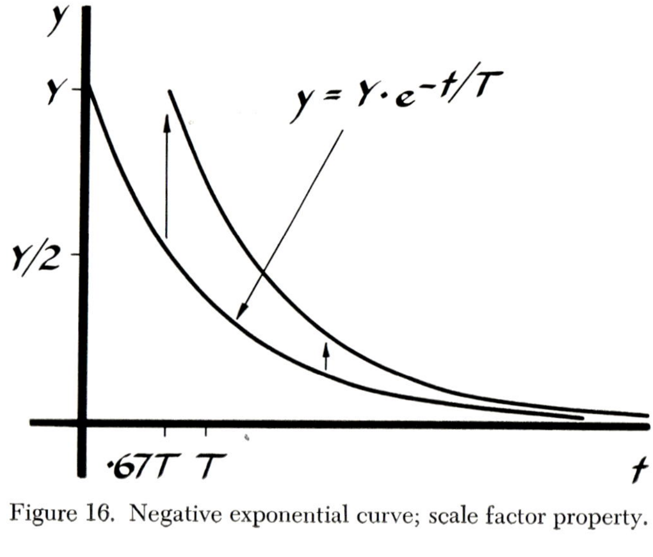

Figure 16. Negative exponential curve; scale factor property.

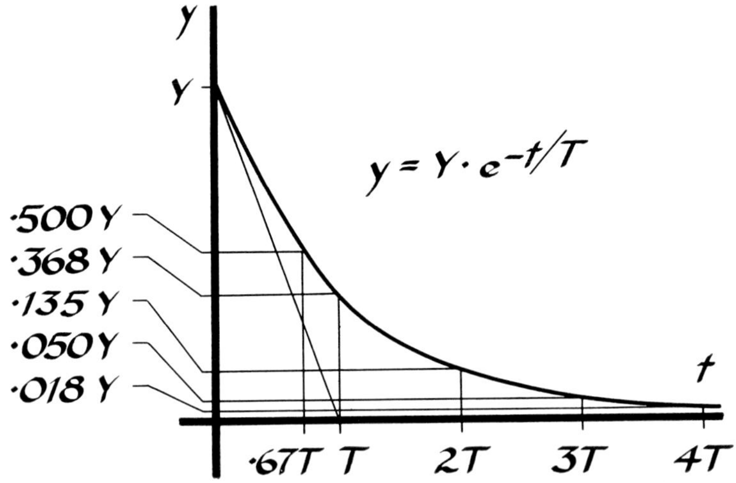

Figure 17. General form of the negative exponential curve.

value, $Y/2$, at $t = 0.67\ T$, restore $y/2$ to its full starting value Y by multiplying by the scale factor of 2. If this scale factor of 2 is multiplied times all the y values for the rest of the negative exponential curve from $t = 0.67\ T$ to $t \rightarrow \infty$ then we obtain a duplicate of the original curve except that it starts at $t = 0.67\ T$ rather than at $t = 0$. The shapes of both curves are identical, and this is what is meant by the statement that one part of the curve, from $t = 0$ to $t \rightarrow \infty$, differs from another part of the curve, from $t = 0.67\ T$ to $t \rightarrow \infty$, only by a scale factor, in this case equal to two.

It should now be apparent that to characterize any negative exponential decay curve, all that is needed is the initial value and the time constant. Figure 17 may therefore be used to approximate any negative exponential decay curve given the initial value and the time constant. For example, when $t = 0.67\ T$ the decay is halfway. The value of $0.67\ T$ is often referred to as the *half life*.

THE SEMILOGARITHMIC PLOT

The general form of the negative exponential function relates y, the dependent variable, as a function of time, t, the independent variable in the equation,

$$y = Y \cdot e^{-t/T},$$

where: Y is the initial value and T the time constant. One of the most useful transformations of this equation is to take natural logarithms of both sides:

$$\ln y = \ln (Y \cdot e^{-t/T}),$$

and from the property that logarithms of multiplied quantities add, write,

$$\ln y = \ln Y + \ln (e^{-t/T}).$$

Recall that the natural logarithm of a number is the exponent of the base e which gives the number and write,

$$\ln y = \ln Y + \left(\frac{-t}{T}\right).$$

Rearranging,

$$\ln y = \left(\frac{-1}{T}\right) \cdot t + \ln Y.$$

Compare this equation with that of a straight line,

$$y = mx + b,$$

where: m is the slope and b the y-intercept; y is the vertical axis, the dependent variable, and x is the horizontal axis, the independent variable. The comparison shows that plotting $\ln y$ as the vertical axis, and t as the horizontal axis, will yield a straight line with slope $-1/T$, and an intercept with the vertical axis of $\ln Y$. Since only one axis is logarithmic the graph is called a semilogarithmic plot, and Figure 18 shows the general case. Semilog graph paper is available, so that the plot may be made directly from the original data without having to convert them to logarithms.

The semilogarithmic plot is useful because it is easier to draw and recognize a straight line than it is a negative exponential curve. Experimental data may therefore be identified as belonging to a negative exponential process by plotting them logarithmically and obtaining a straight line. The time constant may be found from the slope of the semilogarithmic plot, thereby using all of the data to fit the straight line, and determine the

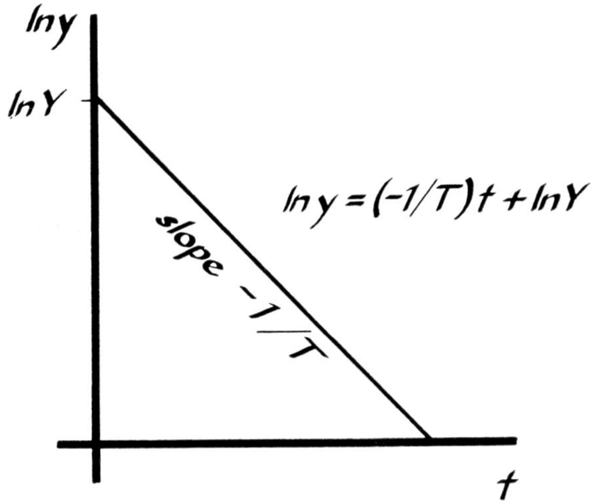

Figure 18. Semilogarithmic plot of the negative exponential curve.

time constant. When data from anaesthetic washout experiments are plotted on semilog graph paper, the plot often takes the form of several straight line segments of different slope rather than a single straight line. The line segments with different slopes indicate that the anaesthetic is being cleared from several tissue compartments, each with a different time constant. The graph is made up of the sum of all the compartment lines, so the time constant for each compartment may be determined by a process of sequential subtraction (starting with the longest time constant) from the original data, known as peeling.

DIFFERENTIATION AND INTEGRATION

The differentiation and integration formulas for the negative exponential function, are, upon inspection, intriguing in their simplicity.

For,

$$y = Y \cdot e^{-t/T},$$

$$\frac{dy}{dt} = \frac{Y \cdot e^{-t/T}}{-T},$$

and

$$\int y \cdot dt = Y \cdot e^{-t/T} \cdot (-T) + C$$

To differentiate with respect to time simply divide the original function by $-T$, and to integrate just multiply the original function by $-T$ and add a constant of integration, C.

The integration of the negative exponential function from $t = 0$ to $t \rightarrow \infty$ is as follows:

$$\begin{aligned} {}_0\!\int^{\infty} (Y \cdot e^{-t/T})\, dt &= [-T \cdot Y \cdot e^{-t/T}]_0^{\infty} \\ &= (-T \cdot Y \cdot e^{-\infty/T}) - (-T \cdot Y \cdot e^{-0/T}) \\ &= -T \cdot Y(e^{-\infty} - e^{-0}) \\ &= -T \cdot Y\,(0 - 1) \\ &= T \cdot Y \end{aligned}$$

From the integration we conclude that the area beneath a negative exponential curve from time zero to infinity is equal to the product of the time constant and the initial value. Figure 19 illustrates this conclusion. The cross hatched rectangular area T by Y equals the stippled area beneath the curve. Because one part of an exponential curve differs from any other part only by a scaling factor, so do the areas differ only by the same scaling factor. Therefore, the area beneath an exponential decay curve from any chosen time to infinity is the product of the y-value at the chosen point in time, times the time constant, T.

The computers available for cardiac output determination by

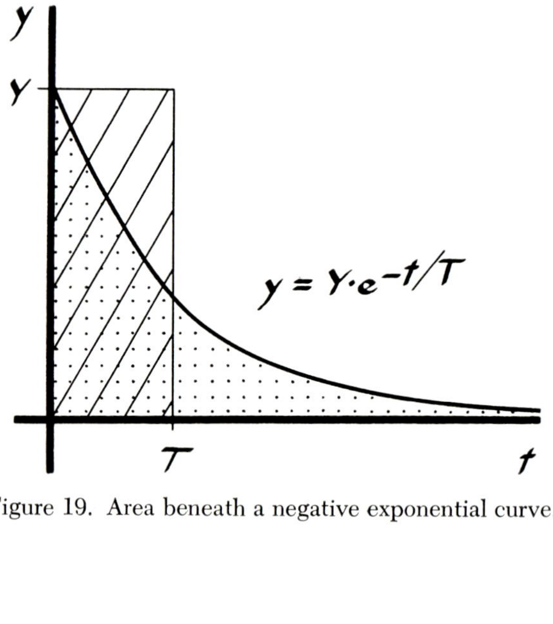

Figure 19. Area beneath a negative exponential curve.

the dye dilution technique use this integration principle to eliminate the recirculation peak. An electronic integrator calculates the area beneath the dye concentration versus time curve up to the point at which the exponential decay starts. The dye concentration at this time multiplied by the time constant of the exponential decay, which occurs before recirculation, yields the rest of the area beneath the dye dilution curve without the recirculation peak.

THE EXPONENTIAL RISE CURVE

To complete this examination of the negative exponential curve we must consider the inverted form of the exponential decay, that is the exponential rise or wash-in curve pictured in Figure 20.

Virtually all of the previous arguments apply with minor adaptations to the exponential rise function because it is simply an exponential decay curve turned upside down. Instead of starting at an initial value and decaying to zero as time goes on, the exponential rise curve starts at zero and rises to a final value as time goes on. The general form of the exponential rise function relates y, the dependent variable, as a function of time, t, the independent variable in the equation:

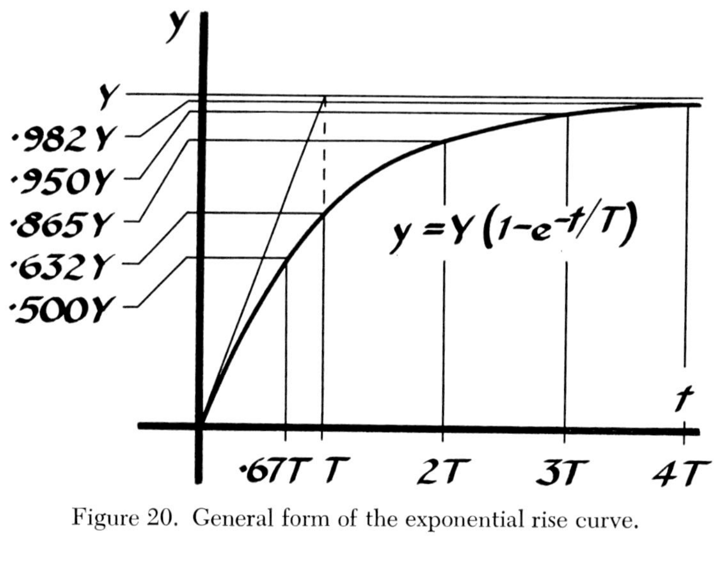

Figure 20. General form of the exponential rise curve.

$$y = Y(1 - e^{-t/T}),$$

or

$$Y - y = Y \cdot e^{-t/T},$$

where: Y is the final value and T the time constant.

The exponential rise function applies to the absorption and distribution of drugs and anaesthetics, the inflation of the lungs at constant pressure, and the changes in arterial Pco_2 and Po_2 after step changes in ventilation, as well as many other aspects of anaesthesia. Figure 20 may be used to approximate any exponential rise curve given the final value and the time constant.

VENTILATORS

Ventilation of the lungs may be carried out by the application of an intermittent, positive pressure to the patient's upper airway (I.P.P.V.) or by the application of an intermittent, negative pressure to the outside of the patient's thorax. The former type of automatic ventilator is most frequently used by the anaesthetist and may be classified as to whether a constant flow is delivered or a constant pressure is applied to the airway. These ideal ventilators are called the *constant flow generator* and *constant pressure generator* respectively. They are *ideal* in that they may be specified exactly.

The basic mechanical forms of these generators are some type of bellows or piston and cylinder arrangement; the bellows are driven either by the force of a fixed weight or spring to make a constant pressure generator, or are driven by the force of a crank arm rotating at a fixed speed to make a constant flow generator. The two classes of generator can also be made from a source of high pressure gas: a constant pressure generator by applying the high pressure through a regulator, and a constant flow generator by applying the high pressure through a very large flow resistance.

All of these real generators have some defects that cause their performance to depart from the ideal. Regulators are not perfect and do not supply constant pressure independent of flow. The internal compliance of many ventilators is high enough to cause wide deviations from ideal performance. The rotating crank driven bellows will produce an output varying sinusoidally rather than a constant flow, although this departure from the ideal may be desirable. Despite these and other differences between the real and ideal, it is both convenient and useful to classify ventilators into the two ideal types because we can analyse, and therefore characterize, the performance of each type.

The termination of the inspiratory phase of automatic ventilators may be brought about by the passage of a preset period of time (time cycled), applicable to both classes of generator, the passage of a preset volume (volume cycled), also applicable to both classes of generator, or the achievement of a preset pressure (pressure cycled), applicable only to flow generators. The expiratory phase is analogous to the inspiratory phase and may be passive or assisted by either generator so that its termination may be controlled by the same methods.

The ventilator is connected to the lungs by an airway and the tracheobronchial tree which offer a resistance to gas flow. The lungs and thorax constitute a compliance at the end of the flow resistance so that the ventilator sees the patient as a resistance leading to a compliance. Such a view of the patient is the simplest model; the real situation is much more complex. However, even such a simple model is complicated by the fact that the values of the resistance and compliance are functions of time and therefore, not constant. If we may assume that the resistance and compliance are parameters, constant for a particular time and patient, then it is possible to describe ventilation by both classes of ideal generator with simple differential equations. The solution of these equations, using the techniques previously discussed, will provide a description of the operation and performance of the flow generator and the pressure generator, ideal ventilators.

The Constant Flow Generator

Examples of real constant flow generators are the Bird ventilator, without the air mix venturi, and the Air-Shields Ventimeter. An ideal constant flow generator delivers a preset constant flow *(F)* regardless of the values of airway resistance *(R)* and total compliance *(C)*. The flow gives rise to a mouth pressure *(Pm)* which differs from the pressure in the lungs *(Pl)* by an amount *Pr*, the pressure across the airway resistance, so we may write.

$$Pm = Pr + Pl.$$

But what are *Pr* and *Pl* in terms of other quantities? If flow *F* is assumed to be laminar then,

$$Pr = F \cdot R$$

The derivation of this relationship is given in Chapter 10, together with other restrictions on its use. Note that the equation is analogous to Ohm's law described in Chapter 11.

From the definition of compliance, *C*, we know that,

$$C = \frac{V}{Pl},$$

and

$$Pl = \frac{V}{C},$$

where: *V* is the increase in the volume of the lungs above the resting volume.

Now, volume is related to flow, *F*, because it is the integral of flow with respect to time *t;* so,

$$V = \int F \cdot dt.$$

In this case flow is constant, and using the integration formula for a constant we get

$$V = \int F \cdot dt = \mathrm{F} \cdot t + C_1,$$

where: C_1 is the constant of integration, and may be evaluated from the boundary condition that at $t = 0$ the volume of the lungs has not increased above its resting value so that $V = 0$. Substitute these values in the equation above to get

$$0 = F \cdot 0 + C_1,$$

and therefore,

$$C_1 = 0.$$

Since the constant of integration is zero,

$$V = F \cdot t;$$

so that,

$$Pl = \frac{F \cdot t}{C}.$$

Now,

$$Pm = Pl + Pr,$$

and

$$Pm = \frac{F \cdot t}{C} + F \cdot R.$$

We have now obtained the equations of interest for mouth pressure *(Pm)* and lung volume increase *(V)* as functions of time *(t)*, constant flow *(F)* and the system parameters, airway resistance *(R)* and total compliance *(C)*. Figure 21 shows these relationships graphically.

The conclusions drawn from this analysis are as follows: Lung volume increases linearly with time from the resting lung volume at a rate (slope) equal to the preset constant flow; the pressure at the mouth increases linearly with time from a value equal to the product of airway resistance times flow, at a rate

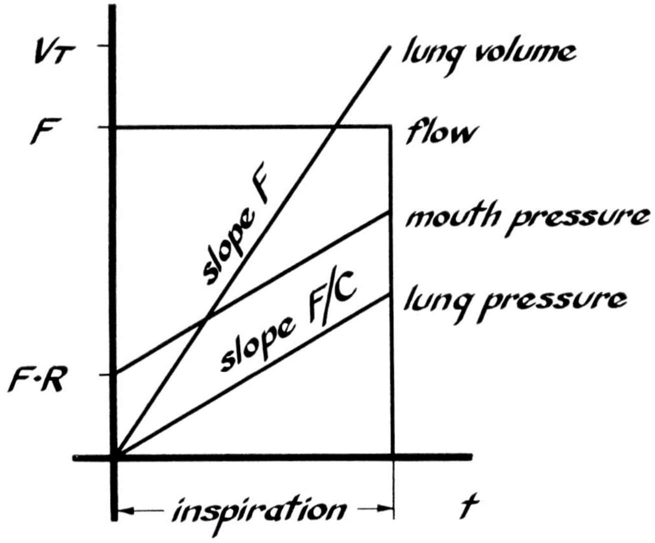

Figure 21. Performance of a constant flow generator ventilator during inspiration.

(slope) equal to flow divided by compliance; the pressure in the lungs increases at the same rate as mouth pressure but starts at zero (this difference between mouth pressure and lung pressure, due to airway resistance, remains constant at a value equal to flow times airway resistance); the volume delivered is independent of resistance and compliance but the generator must be limited in the pressure that it can exert so as not to cause tissue damage.

The Constant Pressure Generator

Examples of real constant pressure generators are the East Radcliffe PNA 1, the Manly, and the Bennett BA-4 ventilators. An ideal constant pressure generator delivers a preset pressure (Pm) regardless of the values of airway resistance (R) and total compliance (C). The resulting flow (F) gives rise to a pressure difference (Pr) across the airway resistance, and a pressure in the lungs (Pl) which sum to equal the mouth pressure.

$$Pm = Pr + Pl$$

If flow, F, is assumed to be laminar then,

$$Pr = F \cdot R,$$

and,

$$F = \frac{Pr}{R}.$$

We also know that flow is the derivative of volume, V, with respect to time, t.

$$F = \frac{dV}{dt}$$

From the definition of compliance, C,

$$C = \frac{V}{Pl}$$

and,

$$V = C \cdot Pl.$$

Now differentiate with respect to time to obtain dV/dt, by using the formula for the differentiation of a constant times a variable; C is the constant and Pl the variable.

$$\frac{dV}{dt} = \frac{d\ (C \cdot Pl)}{dt}$$

$$F = \frac{dV}{dt} = C\left(\frac{dPl}{dt}\right)$$

But,

$$F = \frac{Pr}{R}$$

Therefore,

$$\frac{Pr}{R} = C\left(\frac{dPl}{dt}\right).$$

We now have two dependent variables, Pr and Pl, in one differential equation with parameters R and C and the independent variable time, t. In order to solve for two unknown variables we require two equations. The other relationship between these two variables is the first equation listed,

$$Pm = Pr + Pl,$$

or

$$Pr = Pm - Pl.$$

Substitute Pm-Pl for Pr in the differential equation to get,

$$\frac{(Pm - Pl)}{R} = C\left(\frac{dPl}{dt}\right)$$

Since Pm is constant we now have one equation in one unknown (Pl) and can solve the differential equation for Pl by the classical method. However, there is one more substitution to be made before proceeding with the solution.

The derivative of the difference between two variables with respect to time is equal to the difference between the derivatives for each variable with respect to time. In our case,

$$\frac{d\ (Pm - Pl)}{dt} = \frac{dPm}{dt} - \frac{dPl}{dt}.$$

But Pm is a constant and the derivative of a constant with respect to time is zero so that,

$$\frac{d\ (Pm - Pl)}{dt} = 0 - \frac{dPl}{dt},$$

and,

$$\frac{dPl}{dt} = -\frac{d\ (Pm - Pl)}{dt}.$$

Substitute for dPl/dt in the differential equation,

$$\frac{(Pm - Pl)}{R} = C\left(\frac{dPl}{dt}\right),$$

to get,

$$\frac{(Pm - Pl)}{R} = C\left(\frac{-d\ (Pm - Pl)}{dt}\right),$$

and

$$\frac{(Pm - Pl)}{R} = -C\left(\frac{d\ (Pm - Pl)}{dt}\right).$$

Note that the equation in this form relates a negative derivative of *Pm-Pl* with respect to time, and *Pm-Pl;* that is, the negative derivative of the quantity is proportional to the quantity. Therefore, we expect that the variation of *Pm-Pl* with time will prove to be a negative exponential curve, and that the method of solving the differential equation will be similar to that discussed in Chapter 2.

Now, cross multiply, that is multiply both sides of the equation by $-dt/C \cdot (Pm - Pl)$ to get:

$$\frac{(Pm - Pl)}{R} \cdot \left(\frac{-dt}{C \cdot (Pm - Pl)}\right) = \left(\frac{-C \cdot d\ (Pm - Pl)}{dt}\right) \cdot \left(\frac{-dt}{C \cdot d\ (Pm - Pl)}\right),$$

and

$$\frac{-dt}{RC} = \frac{d\ (Pm - Pl)}{(Pm - Pl)};$$

that is,

$$\frac{d\ (Pm - Pl)}{(Pm - Pl)} = -\frac{dt}{RC}.$$

This differential equation can now be solved by integrating both sides using the following integration formulas:

for

$$y = \frac{1}{x};\ \int y \cdot dx = \ln y + C_1$$

for

$$y = K;\ \int y \cdot dx = K \cdot x + C_2$$

where K is a constant, and C_1 and C_2 are integration constants.

Continuing,

$$\int \frac{d\ (Pm - Pl)}{(Pm - Pl)} = \int \frac{-dt}{R \cdot C}$$

Integrating,

$$\ln\ (Pm - Pl) + C_1 = -\frac{t}{RC} + C_2,$$

and,

$$\ln\ (Pm - Pl) = -\left(\frac{1}{RC}\right) \cdot t + (C_2 - C_1).$$

From the definition of natural logarithms; since the natural logarithm of $(Pm - Pl)$ is equal to $-(1/RC) \cdot t + (C_2 - C_1)$, then $-(1/RC) \cdot t + (C_2 - C_1)$ is the exponent of e which will give $(Pm - Pl)$. Therefore,

$$Pm - Pl = e^{-(1/RC) \cdot t + (C_2 - C_1)},$$

and since the exponents of products with the same base add; then,

$$Pm - Pl = e^{-t/RC} \cdot e^{(C_2 - C_1)}.$$

The constant, $e^{(C_2 - C_1)}$, may be evaluated from the boundary condition that at $t = 0$, Pl is also zero and Pm is constant at its preset value. Substituting these values in the equation above gives,

$$Pm - 0 = e^{-0/RC} \cdot e^{(C_2 - C_1)},$$

and since

$$e^0 = e^{1-1} = e/e = 1$$

therefore,

$$Pm = e^{(C_2 - C_1)},$$

and the constant $e^{(C_2 - C_1)}$ is equal to the pre-set constant pressure, Pm. The final equation is thus the exponential decay curve that we anticipated,

$$Pm - Pl = Pm \cdot e^{-t/RC},$$

or,

$$Pl = Pm\ (1 - e^{-t/RC}),$$

which states that lung pressure rises exponentially from zero to a final value with a time constant RC. We can obtain a similar relation for the increase in lung volume from its resting value because,

$$V = C \cdot Pl$$

so,

$$V = C \cdot Pm\ (1 - e^{-t/RC}).$$

The increase in lung volume rises exponentially from zero to a final value with a time constant RC. The final values may be found by putting $t = \infty$ in the equations. Since $e^{-\infty}$ is zero then,

$$Pl = Pm\ at\ t = \infty,$$

and

$$V = C \cdot Pm\ at\ t = \infty.$$

We have now obtained the equations for lung volume increase, V, and lung pressure, Pl, as functions of time, t, constant pressure, Pm, and the system parameters, airway resistance, R,

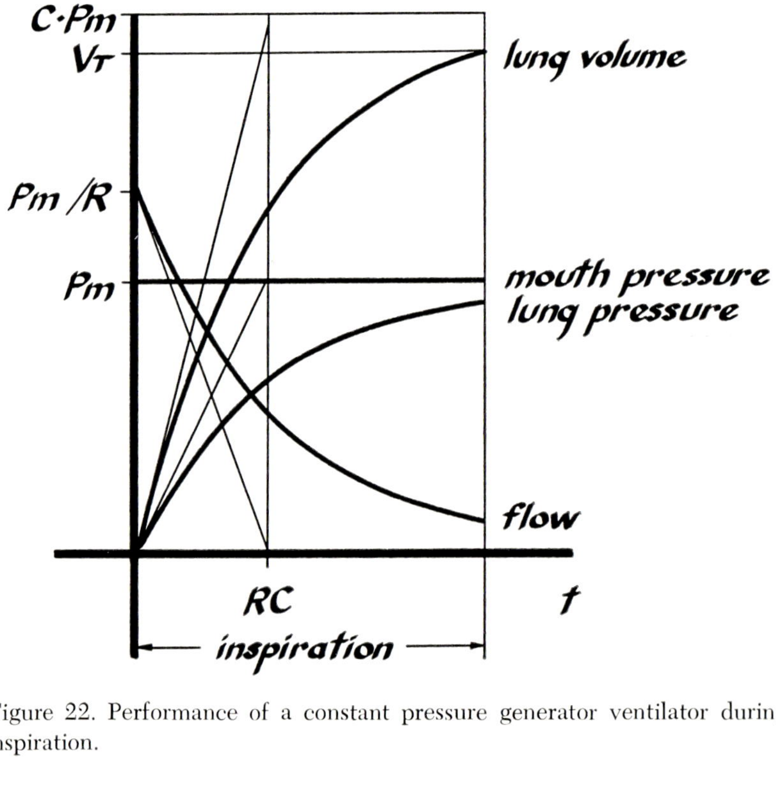

Figure 22. Performance of a constant pressure generator ventilator during inspiration.

and total compliance, *C*. Figure 22 shows these relationships graphically.

The results of the solution indicate that for a constant pressure generator, during inflation, the pressure at the mouth remains constant at the preset value, while the pressure in the lungs rises exponentially with a time constant *RC* from zero towards the value of the mouth pressure. The lung volume rises exponentially with a time constant *RC* from the resting value towards a final value which equals the product of mouth pressure and compliance. The difference between mouth pressure and lung pressure starts at a value equal to the preset mouth pressure, and decays exponentially with a time constant *RC* towards a final value of zero. Flow, equal to this pressure difference divided by resistance, follows the same time course. The constant pressure generator delivers a volume which depends upon the values of airway resistance and total compliance so that changes in these values over a period of time can cause a previously adequate ventilation to become inadequate.

PROBLEM 3

(a) An anaesthetized patient is to be ventilated. His compliance is 50 ml/cm H_2O, and his airway resistance is 10 cm H_2O/litre/second. A constant pressure generator of 10 cm H_2O is applied for 0.5 seconds. What is the increase in lung volume? If the pressure generator is applied for 2.0 seconds, what is the lung volume increase?

(b) A constant flow generator of 250 ml/second is applied for 0.5 seconds. What is the lung volume increase? If the flow generator is applied for 2.0 seconds, what is the increase in lung volume?

(c) Calculate the increase in lung volume if the resistance doubles, for each of the cases above.

Chapter 4

MEASUREMENT AND MECHANICS

THE SYSTEM of rigorously defined mechanical quantities, like force, displacement and power, together with the units in which they are measured, form a means of precise communication of observations. The concepts involved in the definition of mechanical units are not complex so they should present little difficulty for the anaesthetist, other than memory work. They constitute a fundamental vocabulary for the chapters that follow.

THE FUNDAMENTAL QUANTITIES

The three fundamental quantities of mechanics, upon which all the others are based, are *mass*, *length* and *time*. The physical concepts of length and time are readily apparent. Mass, however, is often confused with weight because of the use of similar units in some systems of measurement and because weighing is used as the method of measuring mass.

Mass is the amount of matter in an object, whereas weight is the force of attraction between the object and the earth. Mass is fully described by a number and a unit, for example 5 kilograms, whereas weight requires a direction as well, for example 5 kiloponds, downwards.

Quantities requiring only a number and a unit are called *scalar* quantities, while those requiring a direction in addition, are called *vector* quantities. (Vector quantities are often indicated as arrows on diagrams.) Mass is therefore a scalar quantity while weight is a vector quantity.

Early units of measurement relied on commonly available objects like the hand to measure the height of a horse. Most people's hands are about the same width (4 inches), so the size of a horse could be communicated as so many hands high. More precise measurement necessitated the use of rulers and tape measures that were derived from a single standard length to which manufacturers of tape measures could refer. For example, from 1889 to 1960 the standard metre length was a bar of platinum and iridium kept in the Bureau International des Poids et Mesures at Sèvres, near Paris.

With improving technology, more accurate standards for the basic mechanical quantities have been defined in terms of natural physical constants. The wavelength of the orange light from Krypton-86 in vacuum now serves as a standard for length, while the standard for time is related to the atomic frequency of Caesium-133. In a way it seems as if standards have reverted to commonly available objects again, although the technology necessary to examine these new standards is not so commonly available, and the improvement in precision is vast.

SYSTEMS OF MEASUREMENT

Once the fundamental quantities, mass, length and time have been defined, and units assigned to them, all the rest of the mechanical quantities can be defined in terms of combinations of the three fundamental quantities. For example, area is length times length, that is length squared; volume is length cubed; density is mass per unit volume; speed is length per unit time, and so on. The many quantities defined in this way form a system of units.

Two systems have attained widespread usage: the Imperial System, using the units foot, pound and second and the Système International d'Unités (S.I.), using the units metre, kilogram and second. We shall examine and use S.I. units because they should eventually attain world-wide usage; however, other units traditional to anaesthetic practice, will also be included.

The six fundamental units of the S.I. system, including the three fundamental mechanical units, are listed in Table III with their abbreviations. These units and those derived from them may all be used with the scaling prefixes listed in Table IV with the exception of the kilogram. It already employs the prefix kilo, and so the scaling prefixes must be attached to the original metric unit, the gram.

TABLE III

BASIS S.I. UNITS

Quantity	*S.I. Unit*	*Symbol*
Length	metre	m
Mass	kilogram	kg
Time	second	s
Electric current	ampere	A
Thermodynamic temperature	kelvin	K
Luminous intensity	candela	cd

Table V demonstrates the use of the scaling prefixes and also helps us to visualize the size of some units for length, volume and mass, commonly used in anaesthesia. It is important to note that both the cubic metre for solids, and the litre for fluids are S.I. units of volume but that one cubic metre equals one kilolitre. This equivalence is important because many of the formulas developed in this book that contain a volume term require that the volume be expressed in cubic metres, or alternatively in kilolitres, but not in litres (abbreviated l to avoid confusion with 1, one).

The following sections define the meaning and units of the mechanical quantities, with some applications to anaesthesia.

TABLE IV

SCALING PREFIXES FOR S.I. UNITS

Scaling Factor	*Prefix*	*Symbol*
10^{-12}	pico-	p
10^{-9}	nano-	n
10^{-6}	micro-	μ
10^{-3}	milli-	m
10^{-2}	centi-	c
10^{-1}	deci-	d
10	deka-	da
10^{2}	hecto-	h
10^{3}	kilo-	k
10^{6}	mega-	M
10^{9}	giga-	G
10^{12}	tera-	T

TABLE V

VOLUME-CAPACITY RELATIONSHIPS

Side of Cube	*Volume*	*Fluid Capacity*	*Mass of Water at 4°C*
1 mm	1 mm^3	1 μl	1 mg
1 cm	1 cm^3	1 ml	1 g
10 cm (1 dm)	1000 cm^3 (1 dm^3)	1 l	1 kg
1 m	1 m^3	1 kl	1 Mg

The units for heat, temperature and electrical quantities will be defined in their respective chapters.

DISPLACEMENT, VELOCITY AND ACCELERATION

The term *distance* is readily understood as a measure of the length along a pathway between one point and another. The choice of pathway will determine the distance travelled, as Figure 23 illustrates, so distance is therefore a scalar length. The term *displacement,* however, is used to describe a vector length, i.e. a distance in a particular direction. For example, Figure 23 shows the displacement from point A to point B as the length of the straight line joining the points, with the direction along the line from A to B.

The difference between scalar lengths (distances) and vector lengths (displacements) is carried into the derivative of length with respect to time. The derivative of distance with respect to time is called *speed,* and the derivative of displacement with respect to time is termed *velocity.* Speed is a scalar quantity, but velocity is a vector quantity with the direction of the displacement associated with it. The S.I. units for speed and velocity are metres per second, abbreviated as m/s.

Figure 23. Definition of distance and displacement.

The derivative of velocity with respect to time is called *acceleration.* Since velocity is the derivative of displacement with respect to time, then acceleration is the second derivative of displacement with respect to time, and therefore is a vector quantity with the direction of the displacement associated with it. The S.I. unit of acceleration is metres per second per second or metres per second squared, abbreviated m/s².

The interdependence of displacement, velocity and acceleration can be shown with mathematical statements. Assign the symbols,

s for displacement,
v for velocity,
a for acceleration,
t for time.

Do not confuse *s*, the symbol often used for displacement in mechanics, with s, the abbreviation for second, the unit of time.

$$v = \frac{ds}{dt},$$

and,

$$a = \frac{dv}{dt},$$

so,

$$a = \frac{d\ (ds/dt)}{dt};$$

that is,

$$a = \frac{d^2s}{dt^2}.$$

the second derivative of displacement with respect to time.

FORCE

Force may be defined as the agent which produces the acceleration of an object. When an object is moved, the force required is proportional to the acceleration produced. That is,

$$F \propto a,$$

where: F = force and a = acceleration. The constant of proportionality is the property of the object called mass, M; so,

$$F = Ma.$$

Force is a vector quantity with the direction of the acceleration associated with it. We can determine the S.I. units of force by substituting the known units for mass and acceleration in the equation above. This procedure is known as a *dimensional analysis.*

$$F = Ma,$$

$$F = \text{kg} \cdot \text{m/s}^2.$$

The S.I. units of force are thus, kilogram metres per second squared. This quantity has been named the newton in honour of Sir Isaac Newton (1642-1727), the English mathematician and physicist. It is abbreviated N. One newton of force is therefore the force required to give a mass of one kilogram an acceleration of one metre per second squared.

The defining equation for force may also be written in terms of velocity, since acceleration is the derivative of velocity with respect to time.

$$F = Ma = M \frac{dv}{dt},$$

and if acceleration is constant,

$$F = \frac{Mv}{t}.$$

The quantity Mv is called *momentum.* We appreciate momentum as the difficulty experienced in moving large masses even at very low velocities. For example, it requires much more force to stop an automobile coasting at a low velocity, than it does to stop a small ball travelling at a much greater velocity.

WEIGHT

The gravitational field of the earth causes a freely falling object to accelerate towards the earth's surface with a constant acceleration of 9.81 m/s^2 (32 feet per second squared), which has been given the symbol G. The force of gravity on a kilogram mass is therefore 9.81 newtons. This 9.81 N force is the *weight* of the kilogram mass.

Weight is quite easily determined, but usually we really want to know mass rather than weight. If our weight scale was calibrated correctly in units of force, it would be necessary to divide the weight in newtons by 9.81 in order to find the mass in kilograms because,

$$W = MG,$$

where:

$$W = \text{weight},$$

and so,

$$M = \frac{W}{G}.$$

It is more convenient to calibrate our weight scale in units of N/G. The newton of force divided by 9.81 is called the kilopond force and is the unit of weight with which we usually calibrate our scales. By calibrating our scale in kiloponds, abbreviated Kp, we can read the mass in kilograms directly, since one kilogram weighs one kilopond. An analogous definition in the Imperial System is used to designate the pound mass as weighing one pound force.

PRESSURE

Force distributed over a surface area is called *pressure* and defined as force per unit area, a vector quantity. A dimensional analysis of the defining equation,

$$P = \frac{F}{A},$$

where:

$$P = \text{pressure},$$
$$F = \text{force},$$
$$A = \text{area},$$

will yield the S.I. units of pressure as follows:

$$P = \text{N/m}^2,$$

and since

$$\text{N} = \text{kg} \cdot \text{m/s}^2;$$

then

$$P = \text{kg} \cdot \text{m/s}^2/\text{m}^2,$$

and

$$P = \text{kg/m} \cdot \text{s}^2 \text{ or kg} \cdot \text{m}^{-1} \cdot \text{s}^{-2}$$

The S.I. unit one newton per square metre or one kilogram per metre per second squared has been named the pascal after Blaise Pascal (1623-1662), the French mathematician, philosopher and physicist. It is abbreviated Pa.

Atmospheric pressure or ambient pressure is often used as a zero point in pressure gauges, with positive pressure greater than ambient and negative pressure less. Such pressures are called gauge pressures and the letter g placed after the units; for example, 5 Pa g. The letter a, standing for absolute, is placed after pressures measured with respect to true zero pressure, when it is necessary to distinguish an absolute pressure from a gauge pressure; for example, atmospheric pressure is approximately 10^5 Pa a.

The units for pressure are numerous. As well as the S.I. unit, the pascal, the Imperial System unit, the pound per square inch, abbreviated p.s.i., is still used extensively. Technically, p.s.i. is an incorrect term and the British Standards Institute recommends the use of the pound force per square inch, abbreviated lbf/in^2. Atmospheric pressure is therefore 14.7 lbf/in^2 a.

Other units of pressure used in anaesthesia have been derived from manometric standards. Both the millimetre of mercury, abbreviated mm Hg, and the centimetre of water, cm H_2O, are used as pressure units although they refer to the length of a manometer column. The torricelli, abbreviated Torr, refers to one mm Hg under standard conditions so that changes in mercury density with ambient temperature and pressure are avoided. It is named after Evangelista Torricelli (1608-1641), the Italian mathematician and physicist.

Conversion from manometric units to S.I. units may be found by using the formula developed in Chapter 8:

$$P = \rho G H,$$

where

P = pressure,
ρ = the density of the manometer fluid

(The Greek letter rho is used for density throughout this book.),

G = the acceleration due to gravity,

and

H = the height of the manometer column.

As an example of the use of this formula, convert 10 cm H_2O to pascals. We know,

$$\rho = 10^3 \text{ kg/m}^3 \text{ for water,}$$
$$G = 9.81 \text{ m/s}^2,$$
$$H = 0.1 \text{ m.}$$

Therefore:

$$P = 10^3 \frac{\text{kg}}{\text{m}^3} \times 9.81 \frac{\text{m}}{\text{s}^2} \times 0.1 \text{ m},$$

and

$$P = 981 \text{ kg} \cdot \text{m}^{-1} \cdot \text{s}^{-2};$$

that is,

$$P = 981 \text{ Pa.}$$

Note that the units for each quantity in the formula were S.I. units. By including the units themselves in the formula and dividing out common units the units of the result were determined. (In this case, kg $\cdot$ m^{-1} $\cdot$ s^{-2}, which is known from previous dimensional analysis to be the S.I. pressure unit, the pascal.) The practice of including the units in any calculation will make it easy to find the units of the result.

In countries already using the S.I. system, the pascal is often replaced by the bar. One bar equals 10^5 Pa, approximately one atmosphere. The millibar is a useful size of unit for anaesthetic practice since 1.33 mbar equals 1 mm Hg. Some of the more useful conversion factors between the many different kinds of pressure units are given in Table VI.

Besides manometers, two types of mechanical pressure gauge are used in anaesthetic practice; the Bourdon tube and the diaphragm. The Bourdon tube, shown in Figure 24, is a copper alloy tube of elliptical cross-section, bent in the form of a circle. One end of the tube is fixed, while the other is free to move a pointer. As the pressure inside the tube increases, the elliptical

TABLE VI

CONVERSION FACTORS FOR PRESSURE UNITS

kPa	*m bar*	*mm Hg*	*cm H_2O*	*lbf/in²* (*psi*)	*Atm*
1	10	7.5	10.2	14.5×10^{-2}	9.87×10^{-3}
0.1	1	0.75	1.02	1.45×10^{-2}	0.987×10^{-3}
0.133	1.33	1	1.36	1.93×10^{-2}	1.32×10^{-3}
0.098	0.98	0.736	1	1.42×10^{-2}	0.967×10^{-3}
6.895	68.95	51.7	70.3	1	6.8×10^{-2}
101.33	1013.3	760	1033.6	14.7	1

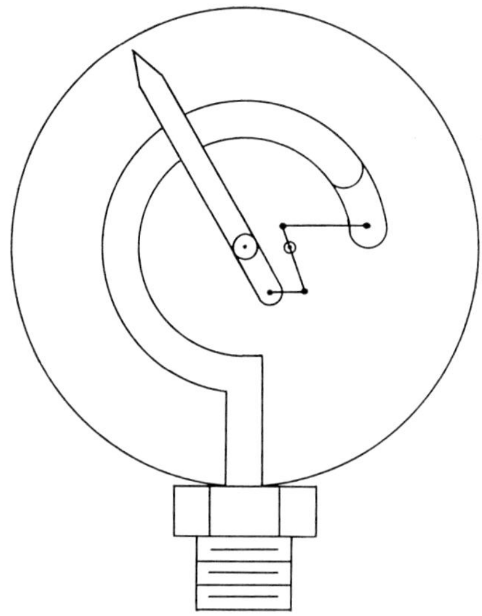

Figure 24. Bourdon pressure gauge.

cross-section tends to become circular, and the free end of the Bourdon tube moves outward, operating the pointer.

In the diaphragm type of pressure gauge, illustrated in Figure 25, a pointer is linked to the centre of a flexible, metal alloy,

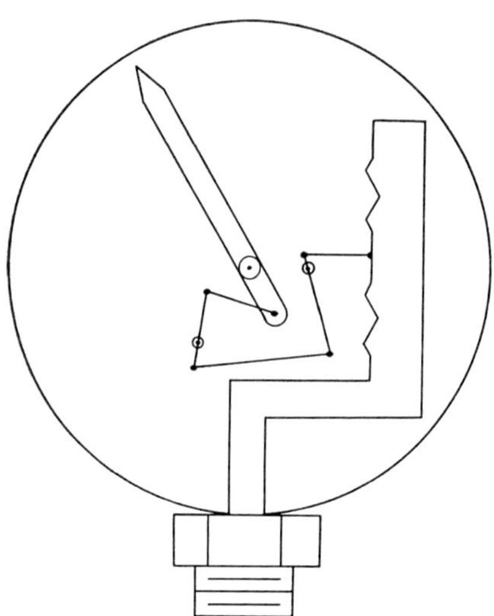

Figure 25. Diaphragm pressure gauge.

corrugated diaphragm. As pressure increases, pushing the diaphragm outwards, the pointer is operated. The scales of these two types of pressure gauges may be calibrated in any of the pressure units desired.

WORK AND ENERGY

Work is done when a force is displaced and is equal to the product of force and displacement:

$$W = Fs,$$

where:

$$W = \text{work},$$
$$F = \text{force},$$
$$s = \text{displacement}.$$

Work is a vector quantity whose direction is that of the displacement. The S.I. units for work can be found from a dimensional analysis of the equation by substituting the S.I. units for force and displacement as follows:

$$W = \text{N} \cdot \text{m},$$

and since,

$$\text{N} = \text{kg} \cdot \text{m/s}^2,$$
$$W = \text{m} \cdot \text{kg} \cdot \text{m/s}^2,$$

and

$$W = \text{kg} \cdot \text{m}^2/\text{s}^2 \text{ or } \text{kg} \cdot \text{m}^2 \cdot \text{s}^{-2}.$$

In the S.I. the newton metre or the kilogram metre squared per second squared has been named the joule, after James Prescott Joule (1818-1889), the English physicist; it is abbreviated J.

Energy is perhaps best defined as the ability to do work. It could also be thought of as stored work, so that work could be thought of as an energy transfer. Because of the interdependence of the two terms, the S.I. unit of energy is therefore joules, the same as the unit of work. The use of the terms work and energy are perhaps best illustrated by considering an actual situation.

Picture a coil spring at rest before it is compressed. If we now compress it a displacement of s metres using an average force of F newtons then the work done on the spring is Fs joules. The spring now possesses more energy, or ability to do work, because by expanding it could push with an average force F while it expanded a displacement s, and so do Fs joules of work. By doing work on the spring in compressing it, we transferred energy to it, and therefore work can be considered as an energy transfer from us who lost the energy to the spring that gained the energy. Conversely, we could think in terms of the spring storing the work that we did on it, ready for release later.

Energy or stored work may exist in many forms, such as chemical, mechanical, atomic, electrical, magnetic and thermal. The S.I. unit of energy, the joule, is used for energy no matter what form it takes. For example, medicine has adopted thermal energy units from heat physics, the calorie and kilocalorie (Calorie with a capital C). These units are equivalent to 4.184 J and 4184 J respectively.

The transfer of energy from one form to another is governed by the law of conservation of energy, which states that in such transfers energy is neither created nor destroyed. In other words, the energy in the universe, or any closed system, is a constant quantity. Many machines and devices for transforming energy from one kind to another appear to contradict this law. For example, the electrical energy input to a ventilator is greater than the mechanical work of breathing done by the ventilator. The "lost" energy is the thermal energy dissipated by friction in the machine. Most energy transformers are therefore qualified by the concept of efficiency:

$$\% \text{ efficiency} = \frac{\text{work output}}{\text{energy input}} \times 100$$

Two types of energy are distinguished in a mechanical system: *kinetic energy* and *potential energy*, abbreviated K.E. and P.E. respectively. They may be defined as follows. K.E. is the energy possessed by an object by virtue of its motion and is equal to the work that was done in producing that motion. P.E. is the energy possessed by an object by virtue of its position in a field such as a gravitational field or by virtue of its configuration (for example expanded lungs) and is equal to the work done in achieving the position or configuration.

POWER

Power is the rate at which work is done (or energy transferred) and is the derivative of work with respect to time. Thus,

$$P = \frac{dW}{dt},$$

where:

$$P = \text{power},$$
$$W = \text{work},$$
$$t = \text{time}.$$

If power is constant, or averaged over a period of time the equation becomes

$$P = \frac{W}{t}.$$

The S.I. units for power can be found from a dimensional analysis of the equation as follows:

$$P = \text{J/s},$$

but

$$\text{J} = \text{kg} \cdot \text{m}^2/\text{s}^2,$$

so,

$$P = \text{kg} \cdot \text{m}^2/\text{s}^2/\text{s},$$

and

$$P = \text{kg} \cdot \text{m}^2/\text{s}^3 \text{ or kg} \cdot \text{m}^2 \cdot \text{s}^{-3}.$$

The joule per second or the kilogram metre squared per second cubed has been named the watt, in honour of James Watt (1736-1819), the Scottish engineer. It is abbreviated W. In general usage, the watt has only been applied to the rate of electrical energy transfer, but in the S.I. it is used for all types of energy transfer rates including heat transfer and mechanical energy transfer rates.

This concludes the definition of the mechanical units. Table VII summarizes the S.I. mechanical units naming the unit for each quantity, the abbreviation, and the dimensional analysis of the quantity in terms of the fundamental quantities, mass, length and time. The remainder of this chapter is concerned with applications of mechanics to anaesthesia.

TABLE VII
S.I. MECHANICAL UNITS

Quantity	*Unit*	*Symbol*	*Dimensional Analysis*
Length	Metre	m	m
Area	Square metre	m^2	m^2
Volume	Cubic metre	m^3	m^3
Fluid capacity	Litre	l	dm^3
Mass	Kilogram	kg	kg
Density	Kilogram per cubic metre	kg/m^3	kg/m^3
Time	Second	s	s
Velocity	Metres per second	m/s	m/s
Acceleration	Metres per second per second	m/s/s	m/s^2
Force	Newton	N	$kg \cdot m/s^2$
Pressure	Pascal	Pa	$kg/m/s^2$
Energy	Joule	J	$kg \cdot m^2/s^2$
Power	Watt	W	$kg \cdot m^2/s^3$

THE WORK OF BREATHING

The actual calculation of the work of breathing in man is a complex problem. However, the type of calculation and application of mechanics to the problem can be demonstrated by considering the simple model of resistance and compliance which was introduced in Chapter 3.

In quiet breathing, when expiration can be assumed to be passive, the following energy transfers occur. During inspiration, the work done by the respiratory muscles results in potential energy storage by the elastic tissues and thermal energy dissipation by the air flow and tissue movement resistances. During expiration, the potential energy stored in the elastic tissues is dissipated as thermal energy by the air flow and tissue movement resistances. The work of breathing is, therefore, the thermal energy lost in the resistances to air flow and tissue movement during inspiration and expiration.

It should be understood that the term resistance, as it is used here in its strict sense, applies only to a thermal energy dissipating element. In a mechanical system such elements are frictional.

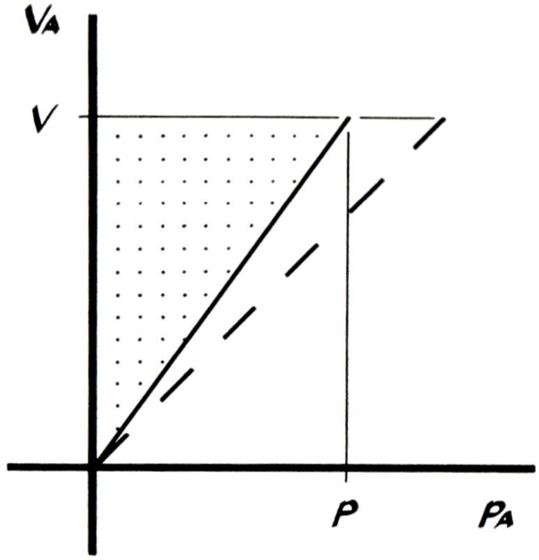

Figure 26. Work of inflating a compliance.

Under this definition, the term elastic resistance is not permissible because the elastic element stores energy rather than dissipating it as thermal energy. These concepts are elaborated in the chapters on fluid flow and electricity.

We can examine the calculation of the work of breathing more easily by considering the inflation of the model lung by positive pressure. Figure 26 shows a plot of lung volume versus alveolar pressure during inflation of the compliance alone. The elastic tissues are stretched during inspiration by a force which starts at zero and rises linearly to a maximum at the end of inspiration, of,

$$F = P \cdot A,$$

where:

F = the maximum force on the elastic tissues,
P = the inflation pressure at the end of inspiration,

and

A = the cross-sectional area over which the pressure applies.

The average force, $\overline{F}$, on the elastic tissues during inspiration is therefore,

$$\overline{F} = \frac{P \cdot A}{2}.$$

The displacement through which this force moves is L, the increase in the length of the elastic tissues, so the work done in stretching the elastic tissues, or the P.E. stored is,

$$\text{P.E.} = W = \overline{F}L,$$

and,

$$\text{P.E.} = \frac{P \cdot A \cdot L}{2}.$$

But $A \cdot L$ is volume, that is the volume increase, V, in the lungs as they are inflated from their resting volume; so,

$$\text{P.E.} = \frac{PV}{2}.$$

This energy is lost as thermal dissipation in the air flow and tissue movement resistances during expiration. Note that P.E. is represented geometrically by the stippled area in Figure 26. The triangular area is equal to half the base times the height which is $PV/2$.

The slope of the volume-pressure line in Figure 26 is total compliance. If the compliance decreases, such as shown by the dashed line, then the area of the triangle increases, i.e. the work of breathing is increased.

The inflation of the lungs through a resistance is shown by Figure 27, a graph of inflation pressure versus volume, and follows a curved path during inspiration rather than the straight line shown in Figure 26, the graph of elastic tissue expansion. The increase in the pressure difference expanding the lungs is due to the resistance to air flow and tissue movement. The increased area of the volume-pressure graph, shown by the stippled area of Figure 27, represents the thermal energy dissipated in these resistances. An increased resistance to air flow bends the curve even further to the right, as shown by the dashed line in Figure 27, so that the area, and therefore the energy dissipation, is increased.

The sum of these two energies, thermal energy dissipation in the resistances during inspiration, and P.E. storage during inspiration constitutes the work of breathing for the model. In Figure 27 the work of breathing is represented geometrically by the total area enclosed by the curve against the volume axis. Using the concept of integration we can, therefore, express the work of breathing as,

$$W = \int P dV,$$

where:

W = the work of breathing,
P = the inflation pressure,
V = the increase in lung volume from the resting volume.

This discussion has simplified the real situation considerably by using a model which assumes that the elastic and resistive properties can be considered as single elements, that is "lumped" rather than distributed in space, and also by assuming a passive expiration. However, the development is sufficiently detailed to demonstrate the increase in the work of breathing with increased resistance and decreased compliance. One further observation should be made. From the previous arguments, and the fact that that resistive dissipation increases with air flow rate, it

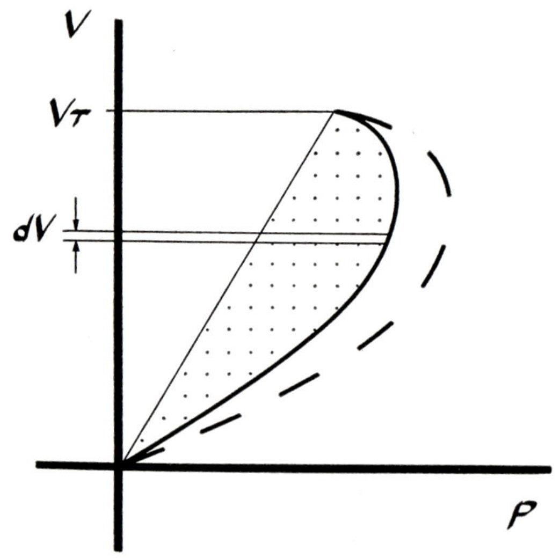

Figure 27. Work of inflating a compliance through a flow resistance.

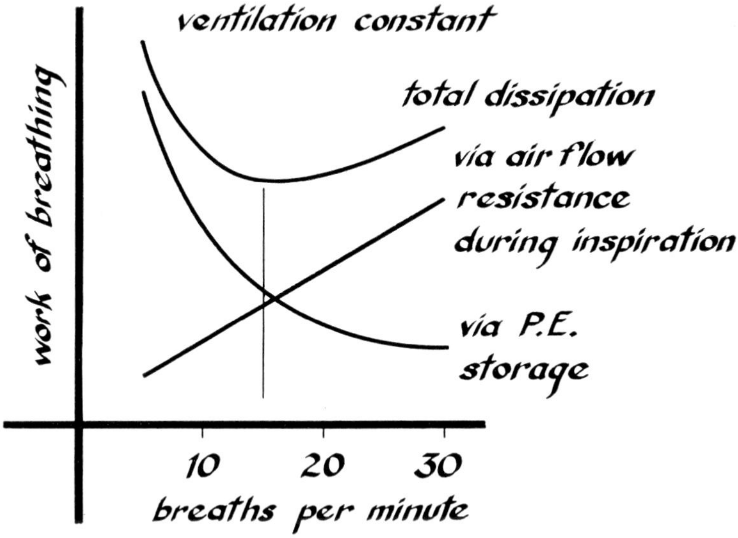

Figure 28. Breathing frequency for minimum work.

can be seen that slow deep inspirations will result in more energy dissipated in expiration via P.E. storage, than by resistance during inspiration. The reverse is true for rapid shallow breathing. These situations are represented in Figure 28. The result is that there exists, for any particular ventilation, an ideal respiratory rate and depth which requires a minimum of work. It is interesting to note that both humans and animals tend towards a respiratory frequency which requires minimum work.

PRESSURE REGULATORS

The pressure regulator, or reducing valve, is used not only to reduce the high pressure in cylinders and lines to a lower pressure but also to provide a constant output pressure regardless of changes in either the inlet pressure or the flow through the valve. Regulators are therefore employed in anaesthetic apparatus to obtain precise control of pressure and flow, as well as to avoid the dangers and expense of high pressure equipment. By means of mechanics we can discover and quantify the operation of pressure regulators.

The internal mechanism of a simple pressure regulator is outlined in Figure 29. The valve and diaphragm to which it is attached are free to move vertically, thereby opening and closing the valve. Spring force, set by the control lever, opens the valve; while output pressure, acting on the diaphragm, closes the valve. An equilibrium or balance of forces is established. A fall in output pressure, due to either decreased inflow or increased outflow, causes the valve to open, thereby restoring the output pressure. Similarly, a rise in output pressure, due to either increased inflow or decreased outflow, causes the valve to close, thereby restoring the output pressure.

If we let p be the low pressure output acting upon the diaphragm of area A, and P be the high pressure input acting upon

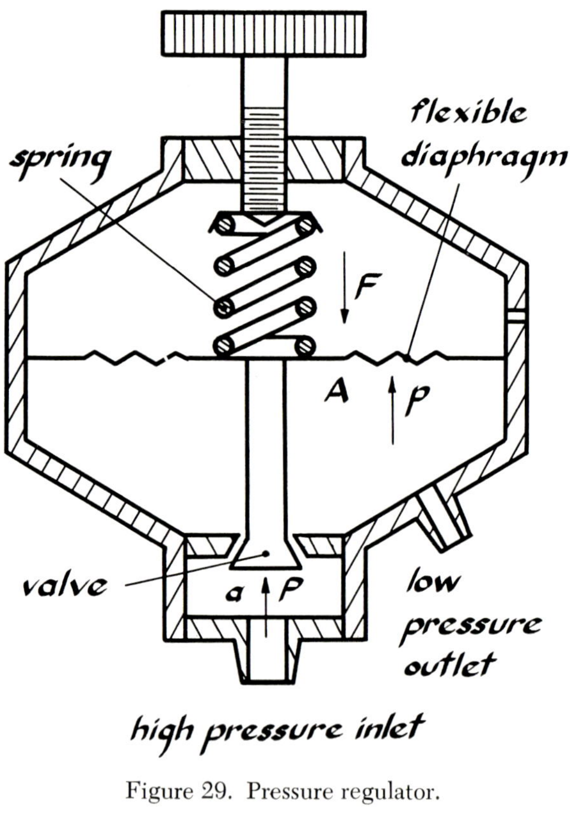

Figure 29. Pressure regulator.

the valve of area a, then the equilibrium between these pressures and the spring force, F, may be written symbolically as,

$$F = pA + Pa.$$

If the area of the valve is extremely small then the term Pa becomes negligible when compared with the other forces involved, and the equation becomes,

$$F \simeq pA,$$

or,

$$p \simeq \frac{F}{A}.$$

For any particular setting of the spring force, F/A is constant, and so the output pressure is approximately constant, independent of flow through the valve, and variations in the high pressure input as long as $P > p$.

Using the complete equilibrium equation we can check the accuracy of the regulation of the low pressure output as follows.

$$F = pA + Pa,$$

or

$$pA = F - Pa.$$

Divide both sides of the equation by A to get,

$$p = \frac{F}{A} - P\left(\frac{a}{A}\right).$$

Suppose that the high pressure input begins at P_1 and falls to P_2. Initially,

$$p_1 = \frac{F}{A} - P_1\left(\frac{a}{A}\right).$$

Finally,

$$p_2 = \frac{F}{A} - P_2\left(\frac{a}{A}\right).$$

The change in the low pressure output is,

$$p_1 - p_2 = \frac{a}{A}(P_2 - P_1).$$

We conclude that the change in the input pressure, $P_2 - P_1$, causes a change in the output pressure, $p_1 - p_2$, but the magnitude of the change is reduced by a factor of (a/A). Note that the change in output pressure is opposite to the change in input pressure, that is as the input pressure falls, the output pressure rises. This situation occurs because the input pressure acts on the valve in opposition to the spring force, effectively reducing it initially. If the valve was constructed such that the input pressure acted on the valve in concert with the spring force the reverse situation would occur, where input and output pressures declined together.

Regulators are made with typical area ratios (a/A) of about 1/200, so that a practical regulator reduces the effect of a variation in input pressure on the output pressure by a factor of 1/200. For example, a change of cylinder pressure of 2,000 lbf/in^2 would cause a change in the output pressure of a regulator of only 10 lbf/in^2.

Regulators are often used to supply a constant pressure to a flow valve and so provide a constant flow for any given flow valve setting. For example, suppose that a regulator connected to a high pressure cylinder supplies a flow valve set to provide a flow F_1 for a pressure p_1. Assuming laminar flow, the resistance of the flow valve is therefore F_1/p_1. As the cylinder pressure declines, the output pressure supplying the flow valve changes to p_2. The flow will change to F_2, equal to $p_2\ (F_1/p_1)$. Expressed algebraically,
initially,

$$F_1 = p_1 \left(\frac{F_1}{p_1}\right)$$

finally,

$$F_2 = p_2 \left(\frac{F_1}{p_1}\right).$$

The change in the flow is,

$$F_1 - F_2 = (p_1 - p_2)\ (F_1/p_1).$$

We conclude that the change in the flow varies directly as the change in pressure and inversely as the initial pressure. Therefore, we can reduce the change in flow by using as high an initial pressure as possible. The limit will be determined by the resistance of the flow valve.

Although the pressure regulator as described is capable of providing pressure regulation sufficient for many applications, nevertheless, in some cases better regulation is required. This goal can be accomplished by connecting two regulators in series (one after another). The overall area ratio then becomes the product of the two individual area ratios, so that the effect of a variation in input pressure on output pressure is reduced by a factor of about $(1/200)(1/200)$ or $1/4 \times 10^4$. For convenience the two regulators are usually housed in one case, and the result is therefore termed a two stage regulator.

The demand regulator is a special version of the two stage regulator. It is designed to supply gas from a high pressure source only upon an inspiratory demand. The output or regulated pressure is, therefore, set slightly below atmospheric pressure so that gas is only released for the small negative gauge pressures that are generated by inspiratory effort. The output stage is designed with a very sensitive response to changes in output pressure so that little inspiratory effort is required to produce a sufficient gas flow.

PROBLEM 4

A man breathes at fifteen breaths per minute. His tidal volume is 500 cm^3, and his compliance is 100 ml/cm H_2O. Convert these quantities to S.I. units, using the fundamental definitions. How much energy in joules is spent stretching the elastic tissues (P.E.) during each breath? during one hour? What is the average power output in watts of his muscles for the above conditions?

Chapter 5

ATOMS AND HEAT

THE ATOMIC THEORY OF MATTER

ATOMIC THEORY assumes that all matter is composed of minute structures called atoms. Visualization of the atom has progressed from the solid sphere of Democritus, through the classical models of Thomson, Rutherford and Bohr, to the almost wholly abstract, modern concept of Schrödinger, Born and Heisenberg.

The classical model of the atom, shown in Figure 30, pictures a massive nucleus of positively charged *protons,* uncharged *neutrons* and other subatomic particles orbited by tiny, negatively charged *electrons,* rather like a minuscule solar system. This model is perhaps of most use, conceptually, to the anaesthetist.

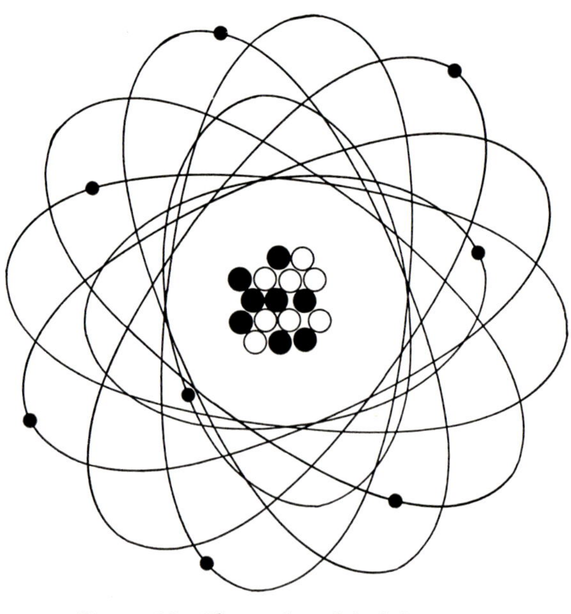

Figure 30. Classical model of the atom.

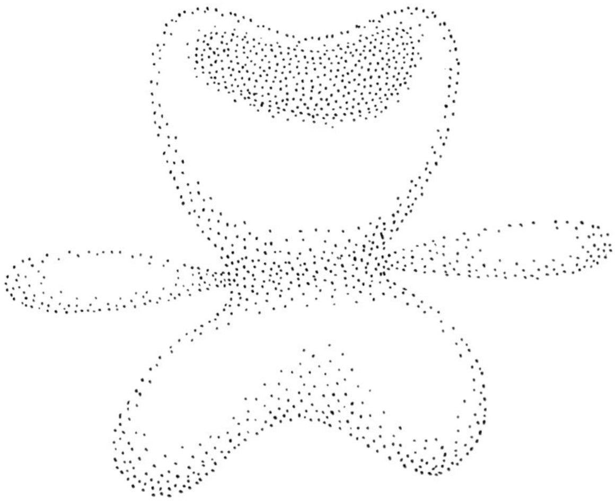

Figure 31. Contemporary model of the atom.

The electron is attracted to the nucleus by a force which increases the closer it gets. Electrons therefore possess more energy the farther away from the nucleus they go, because work was done to tear them away. It is for this reason that we think of the electron orbits as energy levels; the higher the energy level, the farther away from the nucleus the electron. Niels Bohr (1885-1962), the Danish physicist, found that only certain specific energy levels could be occupied by electrons so that electrons could only reach other energy levels (orbits) by acquiring or losing specific, discrete amounts of energy (called quanta). Moreover, the Pauli exclusion principle named after Wolfgang Pauli (1900-1958), the Austro-Swiss physicist, states that only one electron may occupy a particular energy level (quantum state) at any given time. These restrictions are the reason that, as we examine the different kinds of atoms from the smallest to the largest, we find that the number of electrons associated with each atom increases, and their orbital energy levels fill from the lowest, closest to the nucleus, to the highest, farthest from the nucleus.

Modern atomic theory sees the atomic particles according to de Broglie who described them as quanta (bits of energy) with wave-like properties. According to quantum theory and wave mechanics, the position of the electrons and other particles is defined by the Schrödinger wave equation, named after Erwin Schrödinger (1887-1961), the Austrian physicist, which solves to give the most probable position rather than an absolutely determined position. Figure 31 shows the probability of the positions of the atomic particles as an increased density of shading.

ELEMENTS AND ISOTOPES

Although there are a multitude of substances in existence, they may all be broken down into one or more of ninety-two naturally occurring elements. An *element* is a substance composed entirely of atoms with the same *atomic number.* This number is defined as the number of protons in the nucleus and is hence also equal to the number of electrons orbiting the nucleus in an electrically neutral atom. Elements may be further subdivided into isotopes. An *isotope* is a substance composed entirely of atoms with the same *mass number.* This number is defined as the total number of protons and neutrons in the nucleus.

These relationships are perhaps best illustrated by an example. All atoms with six protons in their nucleus, and hence an atomic number of six, are carbon atoms. Carbon is the name of the element. Two of the isotopes of carbon are carbon 12, which has six neutrons in its nucleus, and hence a mass number of 12, and carbon 14, which has eight neutrons in its nucleus, and hence a mass number of 14. The extra neutrons make the carbon 14 isotope unstable, that is radioactive.

As well as an atomic number and chemical name, elements are given an atomic weight. This is a chemical index whose usefulness will become evident later in this chapter. The term weight is misused, however. *Atomic weight* specifies the average atomic mass for an element, relative to a standard average atomic mass for the element carbon chosen as 12. It should be noted that the standard used to be the atomic weight of oxygen, chosen as 16.

By the above definition, atomic weight is a sort of average mass number for an element and will depend upon the proportions of the various isotopes composing an element. The average mass number will, therefore, not be a whole number (unless it is assumed, such as that of the standard), but somewhere between the smallest and largest mass numbers of the isotopes.

In order to appreciate the actual size and mass of atoms, those of the smallest and largest of the natural elements are as follows. Hydrogen has an average mass for its individual atoms of 1.66×10^{-27} kg, and a diameter of 10 nm. Plutonium has an average mass and diameter of 390×10^{-27} kg and 60 nm respectively. Note that the actual mass for an average atom of any element may be obtained by multiplying its atomic weight by the unit atomic mass, 1.66×10^{-27} kg.

ATOMIC BONDS

Atoms react together to form stable complexes called *molecules,* which behave as single units under various physical conditions, and may have properties completely different from their constituent atoms. The strong bonds between atoms are formed by either the exchange or the sharing of electrons in the outer energy levels. Weaker bonds are formed by electrostatic attraction, the force exerted by electrons attracted to spaces containing no electrons. The several types of bonds, and the energy required to break them, are presented in order of strength.

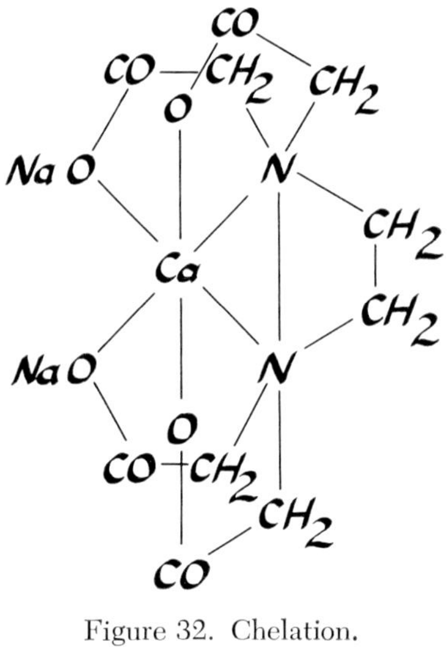

Figure 32. Chelation.

The *covalent bond* is the strongest bond between two atoms, with an energy of about 7×10^{-19} J. It consists of a shared pair of electrons, one donated by each atom. This bond is commonly indicated, in structural formulas, as a bar between the abbreviations for each element. For example, water, H_2O, is indicated structurally as H–O–H. In the *coordinate covalent* bond, both electrons are donated by one atom. The bond is weaker. The formation of several of these bonds to hold a metal ion in a complex ring structure, such as that shown in Figure 32, is called *chelation*. Pharmacologically useful chelating agents like EDTA (ethylenediamine tetraacetate) form several of these bonds to hold metal ions, while biological proteins such as heme and cytochrome C also use several coordinate covalent bonds to hold a ferrous ion.

An *ionic bond* is formed when two ions (an atom with either an excess or deficit of electrons) combine by electrostatic attraction. The ions are formed when one atom donates an electron, thereby becoming a positively charged ion, to another atom, which becomes a negatively charged ion. The energy required to break an ionic bond is approximately 3.5×10^{-20} J. Salt or sodium chloride is an example of a molecule formed by an ionic bond, ($Na^+ Cl^-$). This type of bond, considerably weaker than the covalent bond, is a major component of drug-receptor interaction. Compare the permanent blockade of the alpha receptor site in smooth muscle by phenoxybenzamine, a covalent bond, with

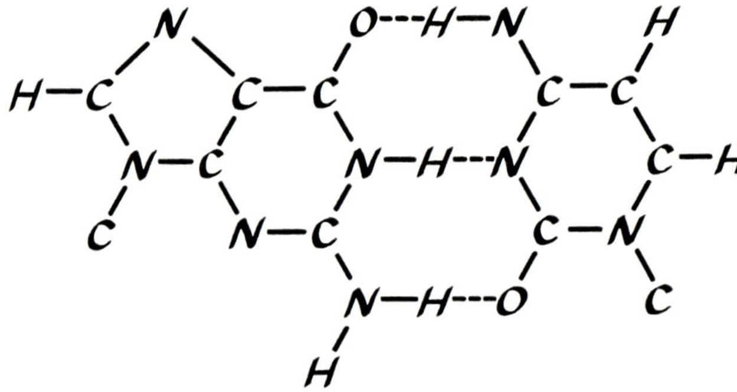

Figure 33. Hydrogen bonding.

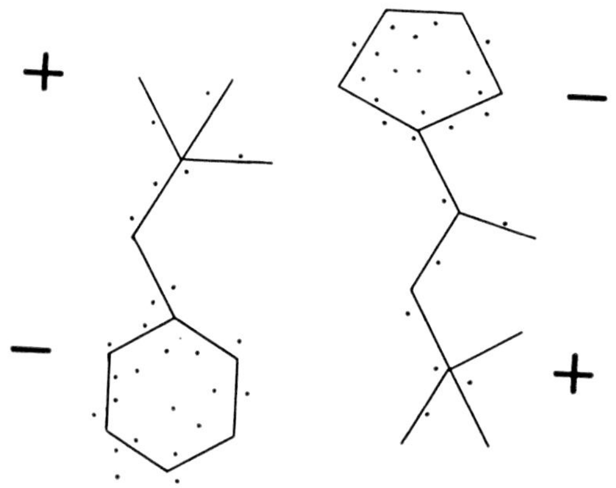

Figure 34. Electron correlation attraction bond.

the transient effect of noradrenaline on the same receptors using ionic and other weak bonds.

The *hydrogen bond* is so called because a hydrogen atom may form a link between two other atoms. The hydrogen atom, in its ionic form H^+, may partially accept an electron from each of two electron donor atoms, such as oxygen and nitrogen, and thereby form a bond between them. Figure 33 illustrates this bond which provides many of the cross links between the complementary base pairs of DNA and other macromolecules to give them their three dimensional, structural shapes. The hydrogen bond is not very strong, from 1.4×10^{-20} to 3.5×10^{-20} joules, and is therefore destroyed by thermal agitation at temperatures over 80°C.

The *electron correlation attraction bond,* known also as the dipole induced, dipole bond and Van der Waals forces, after Johannes Diderik Van der Waals (1837-1923), the Dutch physicist, arises from mutually induced distortions in the electron clouds surrounding large molecules, such as those shown in Figure 34. An electrostatic dipole is formed when electrons gather at one end of a molecule thereby making it negatively charged, leaving a deficit of electrons at the other end of the molecule to make it positively charged. A complementary dipole may be induced in another molecule's cloud of electrons by the attraction between positive and negative charges so that electrostatic attraction holds the two molecules together. While single bonds of this type are very weak, only about 3.5×10^{-21} joules, they may contribute significantly to the attraction of a drug molecule for a receptor surface.

THE MOLE AND AVOGADRO'S CONSTANT

Molecules, in common with atoms, are given a *molecular weight,* which is defined as the sum of the atomic weights of the constituent atoms. Note that the term weight is again misused. The gram molecular weight, called a *mole,* is simply the molecular weight of a substance in grams. The mole is presently in widespread use as a seventh basic S.I. unit, although as yet unofficial. It is abbreviated mol. Table VIII lists the molecular weights of substances of interest to anaesthetists.

By definition, a mole of halothane is 197.5 grams. But how many molecules are there in a mole of halothane? Let the number of molecules in a mole be *No.* The mass of *No* molecules of halothane is therefore 197.5 g. The mass of one molecule, how-

TABLE VIII

MOLECULAR WEIGHTS*

Water	18 · 01534
Oxygen (O_2)	31 · 9988
Carbon Dioxide	44 · 01
Nitrogen (N_2)	28 · 0134
Helium	4 · 0026
Xenon	131 · 30
Nitrous Oxide	44 · 02
Halothane	197 · 39
Methoxyflurane	164 · 97
Diethyl Ether	74 · 12
Cyclopropane	42 · 08
Divinyl Ether	70 · 10
Ethylene	28 · 05
Trichloroethylene	131 · 40
Ethyl Chloride	64 · 52
Chloroform	119 · 38

* P. G. Stecker (Ed.): *The Merck Index.* Merck and Co. Inc., Rahway, New Jersey, U.S.A.

ever, may be found by multiplying the molecular weight by the unit atomic mass, 1.66×10^{-27} kg. So, one molecule has a mass of

$$197.5 \times 1.66 \times 10^{-24} \text{ grams.}$$

Therefore, the number of molecules in a mole is,

$$No = \frac{197.5 \text{ g}}{197.5 \times 1.66 \times 10^{-24} \text{ g}}$$

and,

$$No \sim 6 \times 10^{23}$$

The calculation above demonstrates that the number of molecules in a mole is independent of the type of molecule because the molecular weight is numerically equal to the mole, and therefore cancels out. So, it is inherent in the definition of a mole that one mole of any substance contains the same number of molecules as one mole of any other substance. The number of molecules is approximately 6×10^{23}, the reciprocal of the unit atomic mass, and is known as *Avogadro's constant,* named for Amedeo Avogadro (1776-1856), the Italian physicist. The mole may thus be thought of as the mass in grams of 6×10^{23} molecules of any substance.

THE STATES OF MATTER

Matter exists in the three states shown in Figure 35, *solid, liquid,* and *gaseous,* depending upon the amount of energy and the type of molecules that it contains. In a solid, the molecules are packed in a closely ordered array or lattice. Bonded strongly to one another, the atoms merely oscillate about their fixed positions. A liquid has more energy than its solid counterpart, and the molecules are free to wander throughout the body of the liquid. The bonds between the molecules are fleeting, relatively low energy bonds. They do, however, serve to hold the liquid together somewhat, and give rise to surface tension at the boundary between gases and liquids. The gaseous state is relatively the most energetic state, with the molecules travelling at high speeds, colliding with each other and the walls of the container. The bonds between high velocity gas molecules are insignificant.

If we take a mechanistic view of the molecules of a substance,

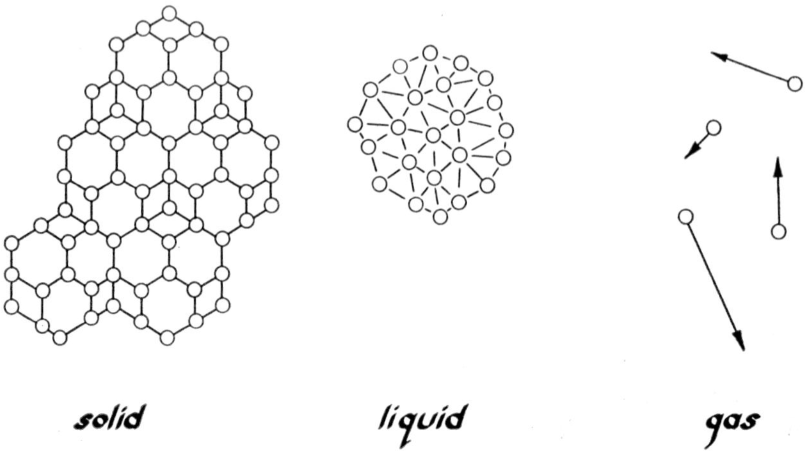

Figure 35. States of matter.

then the energy that it contains will be made up of two types, K.E. and P.E. Kinetic energy, the energy of motion of the molecules is easily understood, but potential energy is not so readily comprehended. Consider two molecules bonded together in the solid state. In order to separate the molecules, as they would be in the liquid state, we must break the bonds. The separated molecules, therefore, possess more energy than the bonded molecules by the amount expended to break the bonds. This energy is stored by the position of the molecules (and is therefore P.E.).

The total energy of a substance in a particular state is thus the sum of its P.E. and K.E. This total energy is called the *internal energy,* which we know more commonly as the heat or thermal energy contained by a substance.

TEMPERATURE

The *temperature* of an object is a measure of the average K.E. possessed by its molecules. Temperature is not, therefore, a measure of the amount of heat energy in an object but the level of K.E.; it shows the thermal potential of one object relative to another. Thermal energy flows from higher temperature objects to lower temperature objects, and so temperature is analogous to pressure in a fluid system and voltage in an electrical system.

Consider a fluid analogy. Two containers, one tall and thin, the other short and fat, are filled with the same amount of water (here analogous to heat). The water level (analogous to temperature) in the tall container is higher than that in the short container. If the two containers were joined by a pipe at their bases, then water (heat) would flow from the tall container to the short container until the water levels (temperatures) equalized. The result would be two containers with the same water level (temperature) but with differing amounts of water (heat).

The S.I. unit of absolute temperature is the kelvin, named for Lord William Thomson Kelvin (1824-1907), the English physicist. It is abbreviated K. Since 0 K corresponds with no molecular motion, the Kelvin scale is not used for everyday purposes. The Celcius temperature scale, named for its inventor Anders Celcius (1701-1744), the Swedish astronomer, is based upon the freezing point of water as zero degrees Celcius (abbreviated °C), and the boiling point of water as 100°C (both measured at one atmosphere pressure) and is much more practical. (The Celcius temperature scale was called the Centigrade scale before 1948.) The kelvin and degree Celcius are units of the same size, only the zero points differ, and

$$0°\text{C} = 273 \text{ K}$$

The Fahrenheit scale of temperature was named for its inventor Gabriel Daniel Fahrenheit (1686-1737), the German physicist and instrument maker. The Fahrenheit scale, abbreviated °F, may still be found and is based upon a scale with a different zero point and different size units than the Celcius and Kelvin scales. Conversion between °F and °C may be made as follows:

$$°\text{F} = \frac{9}{5}\,°\text{C} + 32$$

$$°\text{C} = \frac{5}{9}\,(°\text{F} - 32)$$

Although the sense of touch gives the anaesthetist an estimate of the temperature of an object, it is not sufficiently accurate and precise to be of value in scientific work. The change in some physical property of material which varies with temperature is used for the measurement of temperature. Any instrument that measures temperature is called a *thermometer.* Some of the common physical properties that change with temperature are, the length of a rod, the volume of fluids, the electrical resistance of a wire, and the colour of a lamp filament. All of these changes are utilized in the construction of various types of thermometers.

The liquid in glass thermometer uses the expansion of a liquid, coloured alcohol or mercury, with temperature. The thermometer consists of a thin walled glass bulb connected to a thick walled glass capillary tube; the bulb and tube are evacuated except for the liquid. When the temperature of the thermometer rises, the glass and liquid expand in volume. Since the liquid expands more than the glass, it rises in the capillary.

The volume versus temperature graphs for alcohol, mercury and water are shown in Figure 36. Note that the graphs for mercury and alcohol are linear compared to that for water. The most common thermometer in hospital practice is the mercury in glass type, which, despite its short length of scale and low

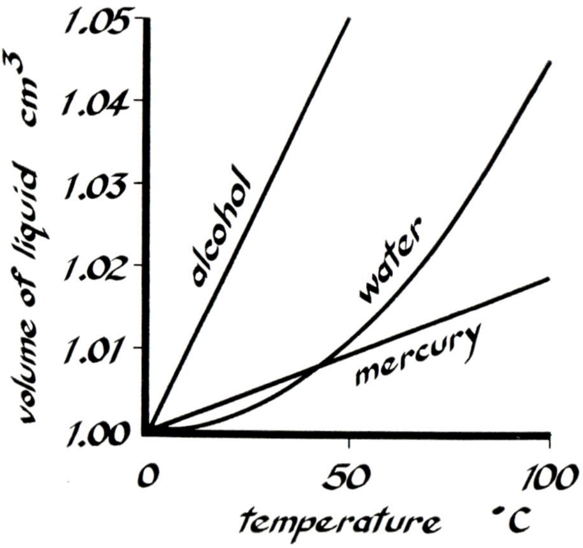

Figure 36. Expansion of alcohol, water and mercury with temperature.

price, can be read with an accuracy of ± 0.2°C. Longer, more accurate mercury thermometers are accepted as calibration standards for most biological research.

The thermocouple is another type of thermometer frequently encountered by anaesthetists. It operates by the Seebeck effect, discovered by Thomas Johann Seebeck (1770-1831), the Russian-German physicist. When two wires made of dissimilar metals are twisted together to form a single loop an electrical current will flow around the loop which is proportional to the difference in temperature between the two junctions. The thermocouple is used as a thermometer by placing one junction in contact with the object whose temperature is to be measured, keeping the other junction at a known constant temperature, and measuring the electrical current generated.

Currently, thermocouples are being superceded by thermistors. The thermistor is a tiny bead of semiconductor material (a heavy metal oxide) whose electrical resistance varies exponentially with temperature. External circuits are used to convert the variation to a linear one so that a useful thermometer is produced.

LATENT HEAT

We have discussed temperature as a measure of the level of K.E. possessed by the molecules of an object and now must consider the other component of internal energy, the P.E. Consider the addition of thermal energy to a block of ice. At −25°C ice has a highly ordered lattice structure held together by various atomic bonds. As the ice is heated, the fixed molecular structure is agitated more and more so that the K.E. increases, i.e. the temperature rises as shown in Figure 37. At 0°C the addition of heat does not cause a rise in K.E. (temperature) but is absorbed as P.E. in breaking the rigid atomic bonding of the crystalline structure of the ice. With further heat added, the ice melts, and the temperature remains constant until all of the ice has become water. The amount of heat required to change the solid to a liquid during the period of constant temperature is called the *latent heat of fusion.* Because the temperature stays constant during melting, ice water at one atmosphere is a stable reference me-

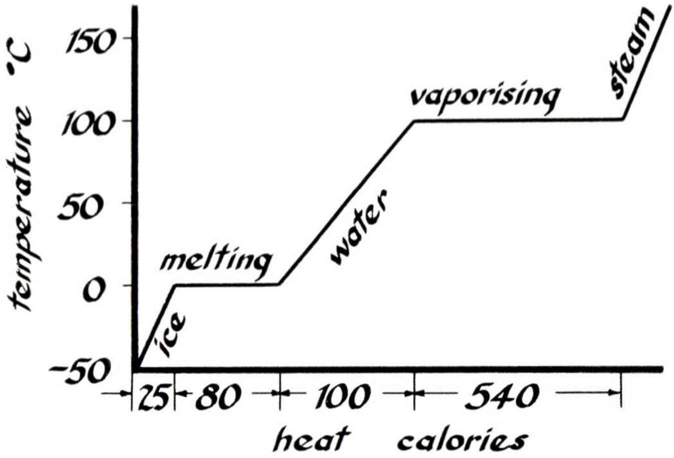

Figure 37. Latent heat of water.

dium, and hence its use to define a point on the temperature scale (273 K and 0°C).

As heat is added to the liquid water, the temperature (K.E.) rises continuously (Figure 37) until the liquid molecules, loosely bonded together, begin to break from the weak bonds, leaving the body of the liquid to become completely free. The water is boiling at 100°C under one atmosphere pressure, and the additional heat is stored as P.E. rather than K.E. The temperature does not rise until all the liquid water becomes water vapour. The heat required to change the liquid into a gas during the period of constant temperature is called the *latent heat of vaporization*. Boiling water at one atmosphere pressure is used to define another point on the temperature scale (100°C and 373 K).

The latent heat of vaporization is an important factor in the design and operation of anaesthetic vaporizers since this thermal energy must be supplied in order to obtain vapour from a liquid. For example, the latent heat of vaporization of ether is 94.4 calories per gram. For every gram of ether liquid converted into vapour, 94.4 calories of thermal energy must be supplied. The latent heat of vaporization of water is considerably higher, 539 cal./g, so humidifiers require heating to produce an adequate quantity of water vapour. With such a large latent heat of vaporization of water, it is easy to understand why sweating is an effective cooling mechanism for the body. Further details about vaporizers and humidifiers will be considered in the chapter on vapours.

HEAT CAPACITY

The unit of heat used in the examples above was the calorie. The S.I. unit of energy, in any form, is the joule; but unfortunately, S.I. units have not attained wide use in heat physics, primarily due to the original conceptual separation of thermal energy and mechanical energy. Anaesthetists are therefore more familiar with the gram-calorie and kilogram-calorie.

One *kilogram-calorie* is defined as the quantity of heat which must be supplied to one kilogram of water to raise its temperature through one Celcius degree, from 14.5°C to 15.5°C (4184 joules). One *gram-calorie* is defined as the quantity of heat which must be supplied to one gram of water to raise its temperature through one Celcius degree, from 14.5°C to 15.5°C (4.184 J). The gram-calorie is often called a calorie while the kilogram-calorie is called a Calorie too, but with a capital C.

Materials differ in the amount of heat or internal energy that they contain per unit mass at any given temperature because their molecules and molecular structures differ. The measure of the ability to hold heat is called the *heat capacity* or *thermal capacity* of the material. Heat capacity is defined as the quantity of heat which can be absorbed by one gram of the substance to yield a temperature rise of one degree Celcius. The temperature rise should not include a change of state. The units of thermal capacity used by anaesthetists are, therefore, calories per gram per degree Celcius, abbreviated cal./g°C. The S.I. units are J/kg · K. Table IX lists some examples of heat capacity.

Because the heat capacity of water is 1 cal./g°C due to the definition of the calorie, the thermal capacity of other substances is often specified as relative to water, and the ratio of the heat capacity of the substance to that of water is known as *specific heat.* Since specific heat is a ratio, there are no units of specific heat; however, specific heat is numerically equal to heat capacity only if the heat capacity is expressed in units of cal./g°C.

TABLE IX

THERMAL CAPACITIES (Cp) @ 25°C, 760 mm Hg*

Substance	*J/Kg · K*	*cal./g · °C*
Water	4184	1.0
Blood	3640	0.87 @ 37°C†
Copper	384 · 9	0.092
Aluminium	899 · 56	0.215
Glass	794 · 96	0.190
Mercury	138 · 9	0.0332
Glycerine	2360	0.564
Ethyl chloride	1130	0.27
Ethylene	1548	0.37
Air	1005	0.24
Oxygen (O_2)	920	0.22
Carbon dioxide	876	0.21
Nitrogen (N_2)	1040	0.25
Nitrous oxide	879	0.21
Helium	5188	1.24

* Ray E. Bolz and George L. Tuve (Eds.): *Handbook of Tables for Applied Engineering Science*, 2nd Edition. Chemical Rubber Company Press, Cleveland, Ohio, U.S.A.

† D. W. Hill: *Physics Applied to Anaesthesia*, 2nd Edition. Butterworths, London, England.

It is difficult to define specific heats for gases because they expand so much when heated. The thermal energy added to a gas may not only be spent increasing the K.E. of its molecules (raising the temperature) but also in doing work on the surroundings, should the gas expand ($W = \int P \cdot dV$). If the volume of the gas is kept constant, however, no external work is done, and all of the added heat is used to increase the K.E. of the gas molecules. The specific heat for constant volume is given the symbol Cv. The specific heat at constant pressure, Cp, is larger by the amount of energy lost doing work as the gas volume expanded at the constant pressure. The ratio, Cp/Cv is given the symbol γ (Greek letter gamma). These ideas are considered in more detail in the next chapter.

The specific heats of gases are very low compared to those for solids and liquids. For example, the specific heats for air at 20°C are:

$$Cp = 0.241 \quad (\text{cal./g°C}),$$
$$Cv = 0.171 \quad (\text{cal./g°C}).$$

Hence, very little heat is needed to change the temperature of gases, and temperature equilibration with their surroundings is very rapid. By the time that air at 37°C has left the airway and travelled through a length of tubing it has equilibrated with room temperature. Such fast equilibration is a major difficulty in the hot water humidification of inspired gases.

In contrast with gases, liquids with high specific heats equilibrate with the temperature of their surroundings very slowly. It is for this reason that water jackets are used to smooth temperature fluctuations in pH electrodes and other constant temperature systems.

HEAT TRANSFER

Thermal energy can be transferred from one point to another in three ways: *conduction, convection* and *radiation.* Conduction is the term used to describe the spread of molecular agitation (K.E.) through a material, convection, the actual movement of heated material, and radiation, the transfer of energy by means of electromagnetic waves such as light.

The conduction of heat occurs as the vibration of the molecules spreads, from the area which is being heated, throughout the material and adjacent substances. Where there are electrons which are relatively free to wander in the lattice structure of solids such as metals, these may spread the molecular agitation more rapidly. The electrons may be thought of as particles which are given a high speed (K.E.) in the heated area, and bounce swiftly into more remote parts of the lattice where they hit molecules, and start the structure shaking. These are the same electrons that conduct electricity. Electrical conductors, like copper, are thus usually good conductors of heat, while electrical insulators are poor conductors of heat.

Since temperature is a measure of the level of K.E., and heat flows from points of high thermal energy to points of low thermal energy, heat flow by conduction is therefore directly proportional to the temperature difference between the two points. The conduction of the thermal agitation will also depend upon the characteristics of the conduction pathway; heat flow varies directly as the cross-sectional area of the pathway, and inversely as the length of the pathway. We can write an equation in words; thus,

$$\text{heat flow} \propto \frac{\text{temperature difference} \times \text{area}}{\text{path length}},$$

and

$$\text{heat flow} = \frac{\text{thermal conductivity} \times \text{temperature difference} \times \text{area}}{\text{path length}},$$

The constant of proportionality, called *thermal conductivity,* is a property of the heat conducting material. If heat flow is expressed in the units calories per second, temperature difference in degrees Celcius, area in square centimetres, and path length in centimetres, then the units of thermal conductivity are cal. cm/s cm^2°C. Examples for three common materials are:

copper	9.2×10^{-1}	cal. cm/s cm^2°C
glass	2.0×10^{-3}	cal. cm/s cm^2°C
air	5.7×10^{-5}	cal. cm/s cm^2°C

The conduction process of heat transfer plays an important role in anaesthetic vaporizers and in heat exchanges for warming or cooling blood. The equation describing conduction heat transfer has a form which will become familiar because it is analogous to the equations describing other processes such as the diffusion of gases through membranes.

The term convection is applied to the transfer of heat by the actual movement of a mass of heated material. The movement may be brought about artificially by pumps or naturally by gravity. In natural convection the mass of fluid (liquid or gas), which is heated, expands so that it is less dense than the surrounding cooler fluid, and therefore it rises. In an enclosed space a circulation of fluid may develop.

Thermal energy may also be transferred in the form of electromagnetic waves. Molecules may become so thermally agitated that the electrons of the constituent atoms are jolted into higher energy orbits. When the electrons fall back to their normal orbits the extra energy is released as quanta of electromagnetic energy. At low temperatures the quanta are small and few so that the radiation is of long wavelength (infrared) and low intensity, but at high temperatures the quantum jumps of the electrons are large and numerous so that the radiation is high energy, short wavelength, visible light.

The loss of heat from an anaesthetized patient occurs by all three processes of heat transfer. Radiation accounts for almost half of the total heat lost. There is also conduction by surfaces in contact with the skin, and both natural and forced convection heat loss. Natural convection of air across exposed skin surfaces, and forced convection of respired air heated by the patient represent a significant heat loss. In addition, the latent heat of vaporization, required to vaporize water so that the alveolar air is fully saturated with water vapour, is lost when the saturated air is expired. As well as keeping the patient covered and the room warm, heat loss may be reduced and even reversed, during anaesthesia, by ventilating with warm moist gases. Therefore, the heat loss from a patient can be markedly affected by the type of anaesthetic circuit used (a closed system loses less heat than an open system), and whether or not humidification is employed.

EXPLOSION HAZARD

In the past, explosive or flammable anaesthetic agents have constituted a major hazard. For this reason, nonflammable agents have been sought and put to use, and a multitude of safety precautions have been used in the operating room. Some flammable agents are still in use, however, and with the use of hyperbaric oxygen, fire and explosion hazards still exist.

On a molecular basis, combustion is a chemical reaction. In the process of oxidation the bond energy of the products is less than the bond energy of the reactants, so the leftover energy is dissipated as heat. In order to induce the initial deformation of the molecules which allows the rearrangements of bonds, activation energy must be supplied, usually in the form of heat. (In biological combustion enzymes supply the necessary deformation rather than heat.)

The process of oxidation may use the oxygen in air, pure oxygen gas or the oxygen in nitrous oxide gas. Nitrous oxide will support combustion almost as well as oxygen because the heat released by the reaction is greater even though the oxygen content per molecule is halved (N_2O, O_2). Nitrous oxide itself is not of course a flammable agent since it is already combined with oxygen.

On a physical basis the process of combustion may be likened to a positive feedback process. Once the activation energy is supplied, the combustion process must feedback enough heat to maintain the combustion or else the process stops. If the rate of liberation of heat is equal to the rate of use of activation energy as fresh mixture is drawn to the process by convection, the flame stands still. If the rate of liberation of heat is larger, then the flame travels through the mixture. With a large positive feedback of heat the flame front travels at high speeds and the pressure cannot equalize quickly so that a shock wave forms which feeds back the heat of adiabatic compression to the combustion process; an explosion occurs. The shock wave can travel at speeds up to 3000 m/sec. (sound 33 m/sec.) with a temperature of 2500 to 3500°C and pressure of 20 to 30 atmospheres.

Flammable anaesthetic agents will burn over a wide range of concentrations although the best composition is a stoichiometric mixture where the concentrations of oxygen and agent are in the same ratio as in the chemical reaction equation. Table X shows the approximate limits of flammability of some anaesthetics.

The activation energy for such mixtures may come from open flames, incandescent surfaces (for example, a light bulb filament), and electrical arcs and static electrical sparks. It takes only about a microjoule to ignite an anaesthetic-oxygen mixture;

TABLE X

LIMITS OF FLAMMABILITY IN AIR, OXYGEN AND NITROUS OXIDE (VOL. %)*

Anaesthetic	*Air*	*Oxygen*	*Nitrous Oxide*
Diethyl ether	1.9-48	2.0-82	1.5-24
Cyclopropane	2.4-10	2.5-60	1.6-30
Ethyl chloride	4.0-15	4.0-67	2.0-33
Ethylene	3.0-28	3.0-80	2.0-40
Divinyl ether	1.7-27	1.8-85	1.4-25

* Coward, H. F. and G. W. Jones: *Limits of Flammability of Gases and Vapours*. U.S. Bureau of Mines Bulletin No. 503, 1952.

a microjoule of heat energy applied to a cubic millimetre of air raises its temperature to 1000°C within a millisecond.

The prevention of electrical ignition, potentially the most difficult to manage, is described in Chapter 12. One obvious precaution against explosions is to air condition, sweeping away accumulations of explosive mixtures.

PROBLEM 5

(a) A blood warming unit for massive transfusion consists of a multichannel bag containing the blood, suspended in a thermostatically controlled water bath with stirring. Blood enters the unit at a flow of 100 ml/min. at 10°C, and leaves at a temperature of 35°C. The water bath temperature is maintained at 40°C. What is the heat flow from the water bath to the blood in calories per second? How could the heat flow be increased (two ways)? What would the power rating of an electrical heater to supply this heat flow be in watts?

Useful information:

heat capacity of whole blood	0.87 cal./g°C
density of whole blood	1.06 g/ml

(b) Compare the heat loss in cal./min. from a patient in saturating the dry gases (0% moisture) administered via Boyle's apparatus with the heat loss from a patient on a circle system where the inspired gas contains 2 percent moisture.

Assume:

inspired gas temperature is 20°C
expired gas temperature is 37°C
respiratory minute volume is 6 litres
expired gas contains 6% moisture

Useful information:

latent heat of vaporization of water = 539 cal./g
1 g of water vaporizes to 1400 ml of water vapour at 37°C.

Chapter 6

GASES

THE KINETIC THEORY OF GASES

According to the kinetic theory of gases, gas molecules behave as if they were small hard spheres travelling at high speeds. Collisions between the molecules themselves and between the molecules and the walls of the container are described as perfectly elastic. The pressure exerted by the gas on the walls of its container is, therefore, due to the continual collisions of a large number of speeding molecules with the walls. Since the speed of an average molecule is proportional to the absolute temperature of the gas, therefore, the pressure of the gas increases with its temperature. If the gas pressure is sufficient, the gas expands into a larger volume.

We conclude that the three quantities: pressure (symbol P), volume (symbol V), and absolute temperature (symbol T); describe the state of a gas, and that they are interrelated. The equation relating these three quantities is known as the *ideal gas law;* so called because only ideal gases behave exactly as the kinetic theory would predict. Real gases approach ideal behaviour only in restricted circumstances, but in enough situations to justify the development and use of the ideal gas law for anaesthetists.

THE IDEAL GAS LAW

Imagine a cube measuring x by x by x, and containing only one molecule of gas bouncing back and forth between two faces of the cube, as pictured in Figure 38. The molecule has a mass M, and a speed between the faces of v. As the molecule strikes one face of the cube its velocity changes from $+v$ to $-v$. The impact is perfectly elastic, so the momentum changes from $+Mv$ to $-Mv$, a total change of $2Mv$. This change in momentum occurs every time that the molecule hits the face of the cube. Since the

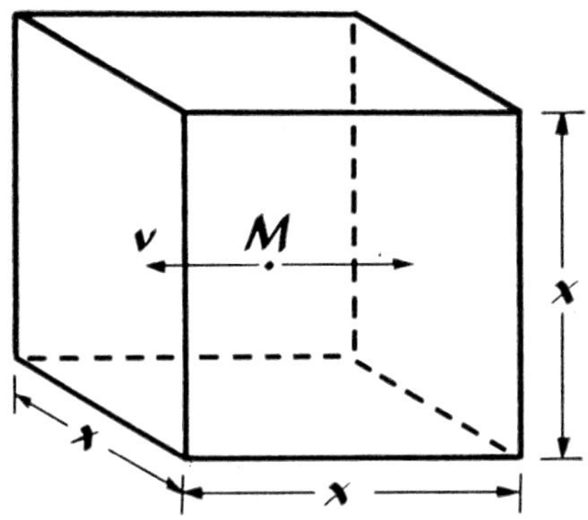

Figure 38. Ideal gas law model.

distance travelled by the molecule, between these collisions with a single face of the cube, is $2x$ and the speed is v, then the time between impacts is

$$t = \frac{2x}{v}.$$

The average rate of change of momentum is thus

$$\frac{2Mv}{t} = \frac{2Mv}{2x/v} = \frac{Mv^2}{x}.$$

Now, recall that a rate of change of momentum is another way of defining force. The average force, F, exerted on one wall of the cube by the bouncing gas molecule is equal to the average rate of change of momentum of the molecule, i.e.

$$F = \frac{Mv^2}{x}.$$

Since the area of a single face of the cube is x^2, then the pressure on one face is

$$P = \frac{F}{x^3} = \frac{Mv^2}{x^2}.$$

But, x^3 is the volume of the cube, so

$$P = \frac{Mv^2}{V}.$$

This is the pressure exerted by the molecule as it bounces back and forth between two faces. If the molecule hits all six faces of the cube then the pressure is one third of the above.

$$P = \frac{Mv^2}{3v},$$

or

$$PV = \frac{Mv^2}{3}$$

From the chapter on mechanics we know that the K.E. of the molecule is $Mv^2/2$, and according to the kinetic theory, the absolute temperature of the gas, T, is proportional to the K.E. We may therefore write the following proportions:

$$\frac{Mv^2}{3} \propto \frac{Mv^2}{2} \propto T,$$

and

$$\frac{Mv^2}{3} = kT,$$

where k is the constant of proportionality and is known as Boltzmann's constant, after Ludwig Boltzmann (1844-1906), the Austrian physicist.

Substituting kT for $Mv^2/3$ into the equation for PV we get

$$PV = kT,$$

and

$$P = \frac{kT}{V}.$$

This is the pressure developed by one molecule of gas. For N molecules the pressure would be N times as great.

$$P = \frac{NkT}{V}.$$

The number of molecules in a mole of gas is Avogadro's number No. If there are n moles of gas then

$$N = n \cdot No,$$

and

$$P = \frac{n \cdot No \cdot k \cdot T}{V}.$$

The product $No \cdot k$ has been named the universal gas constant, since it does not depend upon the type of gas and has been given the symbol R.

$R = No \cdot k = 8.31$ J/mol · K in S.I. units,

and

$R = 62$ mm Hg · litres/mol · K in units more familiar to anaesthetists.

The ideal gas law may, therefore, be stated as

$$PV = nRT,$$

where:

P is the absolute pressure,
V is the volume,
n is the number of moles,
R is the universal gas constant,

and

T is the absolute temperature.

Note that when using the ideal gas law in the form given above, it is necessary to express the quantities in units consistent with those of R. Carrying the units into the calculations will make this necessity apparent.

Providing that the same number of moles of gas are changing from state 1 to state 2, the ideal gas law becomes,

$$P_1V_1 = nRT_1,$$

and

$$P_2V_2 = nRT_2.$$

Therefore

$$\frac{P_1V_1}{T_1} = nR,$$

and

$$\frac{P_2V_2}{T_2} = nR,$$

so that

$$\frac{P_1V_1}{T_1} = \frac{P_2V_2}{T_2}.$$

The ideal gas law stated as above can be used with any units for temperature volume and pressure, including manometric pressure units, as long as the units are absolute, and are the same for state 1 and state 2.

THE LAWS OF BOYLE AND CHARLES

Both of these gas laws are specific cases of the ideal gas law, but whereas the ideal gas law was derived from the kinetic theory of gases, Boyle's and Charles' laws were determined from experimental observations.

Boyle's law, named for its discoverer Robert Boyle (1627-1691), the Irish scientist and philosopher, states that for a given mass of gas, if the temperature is kept constant, the volume varies inversely as the absolute pressure. In symbols,

$$V \propto \frac{1}{P} \quad (T \text{ constant})$$

Charles' law, named for its discoverer Jacques Alexander César Charles (1746-1823), the French physicist, states that for a given mass of gas, if the pressure is kept constant, the volume varies directly as the absolute temperature. In symbols,

$$V \propto T \quad (P \text{ constant})$$

AVOGADRO'S HYPOTHESIS

Avogadro hypothesized that equal volumes of all gases, at the same temperature and pressure, contain an equal number of molecules. This hypothesis is simply a consequence of the ideal gas law. The ideal gas law states that

$$PV = NkT;$$

so that

$$N = \frac{PV}{kT}.$$

None of these symbols depends upon what type of gas is present. If P, V and T are the same for two kinds of gas, then N, the number of molecules, will calculate out to be the same for both gases. To put the idea another way, consider gas 1 and gas 2. Given that,

$$P_1 = P_2,\ V_1 = V_2 \text{ and } T_1 = T_2,$$

then

$$N_1 = \frac{P_1V_1}{kT_1}, \text{ and } N_2 = \frac{P_2V_2}{kT_2}.$$

Therefore

$$N_1 = N_2.$$

A useful corollary of this hypothesis is that one mole of gas, at a specified temperature and pressure, will occupy a particular volume, independent of the type of gas. Using the ideal gas law we can determine that at a standard temperature and pressure of 0°C (273 K) and 760 mm Hg ($\simeq 10^5$ Pa) respectively, one mole of any gas will occupy 22.4 litres. At room temperature (20°C) the volume increases to 24.0 litres, and at body temperature (37°C) to 25.4 litres. The relations are worth memorizing.

DALTON'S LAW OF PARTIAL PRESSURES

In a mixture of gases, the pressure depends only upon the total number of molecules present in the volume, not upon what kind they are. If we removed all of the gases in the mixture but one, then the pressure would be determined by the number of its molecules present in the volume. This pressure, exerted by the one type of gas alone in the volume, is defined as the *partial pressure* for that particular gas. The sum of the partial pressures for each gas in the mixture equals the pressure of the mixture, because the number of molecules of each gas sum to give the total number of molecules producing the pressure.

The argument may also be stated mathematically. Given gases x, y and z, whose molecules number Nx, Ny and Nz respectively, in a volume V at an absolute temperature T, find the total pressure of the mixture, P, in terms of the partial pressures.

$$P = \frac{(Nx + Ny + Nz)\ kT}{V},$$

and

$$P = \frac{Nx \cdot k \cdot T}{V} + \frac{Ny \cdot k \cdot T}{V} + \frac{Nz \cdot k \cdot t}{V}.$$

But, by definition,

$$\frac{Nx \cdot k \cdot T}{V} = Px,$$

$$\frac{Ny \cdot k \cdot T}{V} = Py,$$

and

$$\frac{Nz \cdot k \cdot T}{V} = Pz.$$

Therefore, substituting in the equation for P yields

$$P = Px + Py + Pz.$$

Dalton's law, named after its discoverer John Dalton (1766-1844), the English chemist and physicist, states that the pressure exerted by a mixture of gases is equal to the sum of the partial pressures which each gas would exert if it alone occupied the same space. As a corollary, each constituent gas in a mixture exerts a partial pressure which is the same proportion of the total pressure as its volume is of the total volume, that is

$$Px = \left(\frac{Vx}{V}\right) P = Fx \cdot P,$$

where Vx is the volume occupied by gas x at pressure P, and Fx is the fractional concentration of gas x. Mathematically,

$$P \cdot Vx = Nx \cdot k \cdot T,$$

and

$$Px \cdot V = Nx \cdot k \cdot T.$$

Therefore

$$Px \cdot V = P \cdot Vx,$$

and

$$Px = \left(\frac{Vx}{V}\right) P.$$

The concept of partial pressure helps in many situations of interest to the anaesthetist, for example, the dilution of alveolar oxygen by water vapour. Assuming that the fractional concentration of oxygen in inspired air is 20.93%, then,

$$P\text{I}_{O_2} = 0.2093 \times 760 = 159 \text{ mm Hg},$$

assuming that atmospheric pressure is 760 mm Hg. As the air is inspired, water vapour is added until the alveolar air is fully saturated. The partial pressure of the water vapour in alveolar air is thus, 47 mm Hg. Therefore, the partial pressure of the inspired air is only 760 – 47 = 713 mm Hg in the alveolar air. Now part of the alveolar air mixture, 20.93 percent of the inspired air is oxygen, and so

$$P\text{A}_{O_2} = 0.2093 \times 713 = 149 \text{ mm Hg}.$$

The fractional concentration of oxygen in the alveolar air mixture is less than it was in inspired air.

$$F_{A_{O_2}} = \frac{149}{760} = 0.196 = 19.6\%$$

In other words, additional water vapour in the alveolar air dilutes the fractional concentration of oxygen by an amount proportional to the reduction in the total pressure of the inspired gas mixture, that is

$$F_{A_{O_2}} = 0.2093 \times \frac{(760 - 47)}{760} = 0.196 = 19.6\%$$

Dalton's law, while accurate enough at atmospheric pressure levels, becomes inaccurate at the pressure levels encountered in cylinders because of the compressibility of gases like CO_2 and N_2O at high pressures. For example, a cylinder may contain 5 percent CO_2 95 percent O_2 according to the ratio of the partial pressures (determined as the cylinder was filled) but actually may contain only 4.9 percent CO_2. The CO_2, added first, was compressed by the O_2 as the cylinder was filled. In such cases, the fractional concentrations must be determined from the actual volumes added to the cylinder.

ADIABATIC AND ISOTHERMAL CHANGES IN VOLUME

From the definitions given in Chapter 4, we know that work is measured in the same units as energy, and that we may regard energy as the ability to do work or conversely, work as the transfer of energy. The kinetic theory of gases embodies the concept that the temperature of a gas is a measure of the level of the K.E. possessed by its constituent molecules. This kinetic energy may be thought of in terms of mechanical energy or in terms of heat, interchangeably (the units are the same in the S.I.). However, the actual transfer of energy between these two forms is not so interchangeable. We cannot, unfortunately, convert heat energy into mechanical energy very efficiently, but we can convert mechanical energy into heat all too readily.

With the ideas above in mind, consider the compression and expansion of a volume of gas. The gas volume can be compressed only by doing work on it, that is to say, by transferring energy to it. If energy has been added then the internal energy of the gas must have increased, and the temperature reflecting the level of K.E. must have also increased. The temperature of the compressed gas will now be higher than its surroundings, and so heat will flow from the gas into the environment until the temperatures equalize. When the gas is expanded the processes are reversed. The gas itself does work on its surroundings (equal to the amount of energy given to it during compression), and so its temperature falls. Heat flows back to the gas from its environment until the temperatures equalize.

An *adiabatic process* is defined as the expansion or compression of a gas with no heat energy exchanged with its environment. An *isothermal process* is defined as the compression or expansion of a gas with all the heat exchanged, i.e. at constant temperature. Since heat exchange takes time, real processes will be somewhere in between these two extremes, depending upon the time taken. A rapid change in volume may be thought of as adiabatic and a very slow change in volume as isothermal.

For example, ventilators are often tested on a model compliance made from a large bottle. The inflation should be isothermal like the ventilation of the lungs, but at high cycling rates the expansion and compression of the gas inside the bottle may approach an adiabatic process. Investigators try to achieve an isothermal process by filling the glass bottle with copper wool, a good heat conductor and reservoir.

The rapid release of gas from a high pressure cylinder is a good example of an adiabatic expansion. When the gas is suddenly released from the valve it expands adiabatically; its internal energy falling by an amount equal to the work done to compress it into the cylinder and also equal to the work done by the expanding gas on its surroundings. The expanded gas is cold, and it is therefore important to prevent water from contaminating a compressed gas since ice may form in the valve, obstructing the flow of gas.

In order to quantitate the changes in temperature that may occur in an adiabatic process, recall the definitions of Cv, the specific heat for a gas at constant volume; and of Cp, the specific heat of a gas at constant pressure, which were given in the last chapter. Without stating it then, we used the first law of thermodynamics, a corollary of the law of conservation of energy. The first law of thermodynamics states that when heat is added to a gas, and it expands at a constant pressure, the heat added is equal to the increase in the internal energy of the gas (K.E.) plus the work done by the expanding gas. The law may be stated mathematically by using the differentials of the variables to signify minutely small changes in each variable. Thus,

$$dH = dU + P \cdot dV,$$

where:

dU = the rise in the internal energy of the gas,
dH = the amount of heat added to the gas,
P = the pressure of the gas (constant),

and

dV = the increase in the volume of the gas.

If the gas is not allowed to expand (V constant) then,

$$dH = dU.$$

The definition of the specific heats for an ideal gas is based upon the first law of thermodynamics as stated above; it is illustrated in Figure 39. Note that in both processes dU is the same because the temperature change is the same, and the internal energy change is a function of temperature only, for an ideal gas. (n is the number of moles of gas involved.)

From the definitions in Figure 39:

$$n \cdot Cp \cdot dT = dU + P \cdot dV,$$

and

$$n \cdot Cv \cdot dT = dU$$

Since dU is the same in both equations,

$$n \cdot Cp \cdot dT = n \cdot Cv \cdot dT + P \cdot dV.$$

Now recall the ideal gas law,

$$PV = nRT,$$

and take its differential form for a constant pressure expansion,

$$P \cdot dV = n \cdot R \cdot dT.$$

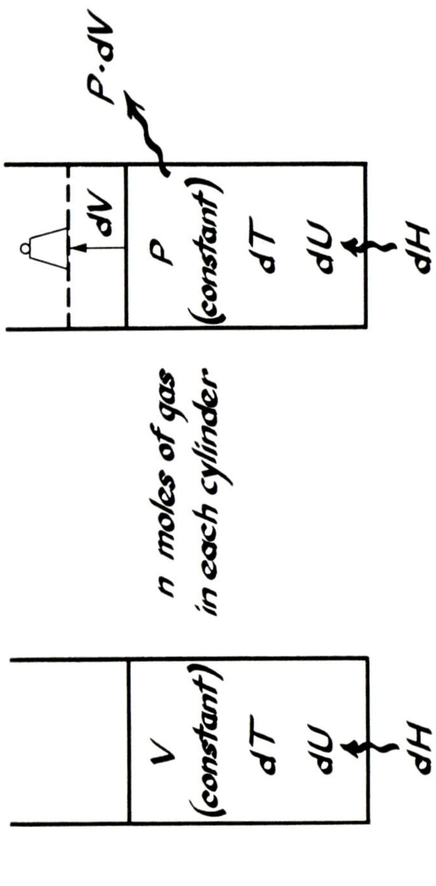

$$C_v = \frac{dH}{dT \cdot n} = \frac{dU}{dT \cdot n} \qquad C_p = \frac{dH}{dT \cdot n} = \frac{dU + P \cdot dV}{dT \cdot n}$$

Figure 39. Specific heats of an ideal gas.

Substituting in the specific heat equation yields,

$$n \cdot Cp \cdot dT = n \cdot Cv \cdot dT + n \cdot R \cdot dT,$$

and dividing both sides by $n \cdot dT$ we get:

$$Cp = Cv + R,$$

or

$$Cp - Cv = R.$$

The above relationship will be useful in the following development of the relation between T and V in an adiabatic process.

The first law of thermodynamics is

$$dH = dU + P \cdot dV.$$

But in an adiabatic process $dH = 0$;

so

$$dU = -P \cdot dV$$

in an adiabatic process. The statement above now says that when a gas expands by a tiny amount dV, at a constant pressure P, then the internal energy decreases by a minute amount dU, equal to the work done by the expanding gas, $P \cdot dV$, as long as no heat is added from the surroundings.

From the definition of the specific heat at constant volume we know that,

$$n \cdot Cv = \frac{dU}{dT}, \text{ and } n \cdot Cv \cdot dT = dU.$$

Therefore, for an adiabatic process,

$$n \cdot Cv \cdot dT = -P \cdot dV,$$

From the ideal gas law,

$$P = \frac{n \cdot R \cdot T}{V},$$

and substituting for P in the adiabatic equation yields

$$n \cdot Cv \cdot dT = -\frac{n \cdot R \cdot T \cdot dV}{V}$$

Dividing both sides of the equation by $n \cdot Cv \cdot T$ we obtain

$$\frac{dT}{T} = -\frac{R}{Cv} \cdot \frac{dV}{V}.$$

Since both R and Cv are constant for any particular gas we have now achieved the desired equation; a quantitative relationship between temperature and volume in an adiabatic process. Although the equation is a differential equation, we can solve it using the classical technique explained in Chapter 2.

Recall that:

for

$$y = \frac{1}{x};\ \int y dx = \ln x + \text{constant},$$

and integrate both sides of the adiabatic equation as follows:

$$\int \frac{dT}{T} = -\frac{R}{Cv} \int \frac{dV}{V},$$

$$\ln T + \text{a constant} = -\frac{R}{Cv} \cdot \ln V + \text{a constant},$$

and

$$\ln T + \frac{R}{Cv} \cdot \ln V = \text{a constant.}$$

From the laws governing the manipulation of logarithms given in Chapter 1, we know that a summation of logarithms is the multiplication of the actual numbers, and that a constant times the logarithm of a number is that number to the power of the constant, so that the adiabatic equation becomes,

$$T \cdot V^{(R/Cv)} = \text{a constant.}$$

From the previous discussion of the specific heats of an ideal gas we know that:

$$Cp - Cv = R.$$

Divide both sides by Cv to get

$$\frac{Cp}{Cv} - 1 = \frac{R}{Cv},$$

and since

$$\frac{Cp}{Cv} = \gamma,$$

therefore

$$\frac{R}{Cv} = \gamma - 1.$$

Substituting in the adiabatic equation yields

$$T \cdot V^{\gamma - 1} = \text{a constant}$$

In its more useful form, applied between states 1 and 2, the adiabatic equation becomes

$$T_1 \cdot V_1^{\gamma - 1} = T_2 \cdot V_2^{\gamma - 1}$$

If we want to know the pressure change as volume changes adiabatically from V_1 to V_2, instead of the temperature change, then we can substitute for T in the equation using the ideal gas law.

$$PV = nRT,$$

and

$$T = \frac{PV}{nR}.$$

Substituting for T in the adiabatic equation yields

$$\frac{PV}{nR} \cdot V^{(\gamma - 1)} = \text{constant},$$

and

$$PV^{\gamma} = \text{a constant} \cdot nR = \text{a constant}.$$

Between states 1 and 2;

$$P_1V_1^{\gamma} = P_2V_2^{\gamma}.$$

Both the pressure and temperature versions of the adiabatic gas law contain exponents which the anaesthetist may find difficult to evaluate without the aid of a slide rule or electronic calculator. The two examples included here show how the adiabatic equations may be solved using log tables.

Suppose that one litre of compressed air at 20°C expands adia-

TABLE XI

RATIOS OF SPECIFIC HEATS FOR GASES (γ)*

Gas	$\gamma = Cp/Cv$
N_2	1.40
O_2	1.40
CO_2	1.30
N_2O	1.31
Air	1.41
He	1.66

* R. E. Bolz and G. L. Tuve (Eds.): *Handbook of Tables for Applied Engineering Science*, 2nd Edition. Chemical Rubber Company Press, Cleveland, Ohio, U.S.A.

batically to two litres. What is the temperature of the expanded gas? γ for air may be obtained from Table XI as 1.41.
For an adiabatic process:

$$T_1V_1^{(\gamma - 1)} = T_2V_2^{(\gamma - 1)}.$$

Solve for T_2,

$$T_2 = \frac{T_1V_1^{(\gamma - 1)}}{V_2^{(\gamma - 1)}} = T_1 \left(\frac{V_1}{V_2}\right)^{\gamma - 1}$$

Now

$$T_1 = 293 \text{ K}; \ \gamma - 1 = 1.41 - 1 = 0.41$$

$$V_1 = 1 \text{ litre}; \ V_2 = 2 \text{ litres}$$

and

$$T_2 = 293(0.5)^{0.41}.$$

The computation may be simplified by writing the equation in logarithmic form.

$$\begin{aligned} \log(T_2) &= \log(293) + 0.41 \log(0.5) \\ \log(293) &= \log(2.93 \times 10^2) = 2 + 0.4669 = 2.4669 \\ 0.41 \log(0.5) &= 0.41 \log(5.0 \times 10^{-1}) = \\ (-1 + 0.699)\ 0.41 &= (-0.301)0.41 = -0.1234 \\ \log(T_2) &= 2.3435 \end{aligned}$$

$$\begin{aligned} T_2 &= \text{antilog } (2 + 0.3435) \\ T_2 &= 10^2 \times 2.206 \\ T_2 &= 220 \text{ K or } -53°\text{C} \end{aligned}$$

The expanded gas reaches a temperature of −53°C if the expansion was adiabatic and shows no change in temperature if the expansion was isothermal.

Suppose that two litres of air at atmospheric pressure are adiabatically compressed to one litre. What is the resulting pressure?

For an adiabatic process: $P_1V_1^{\gamma} = P_2V_2^{\gamma}$.
Solve for P_2,

$$P_2 = \frac{P_1V_1^{\gamma}}{V_2^{\gamma}} = P_1 \left(\frac{V_1}{V_2}\right)^{\gamma}$$

Now,

$$P_1 = 1 \text{ atmosphere}; \quad \gamma = 1.41$$

$$V_1 = 2 \text{ litres}; \quad V_2 = 1 \text{ litre}$$

and

$$P_2 = 1 \times (2)^{1.41}.$$

The computation may be simplified by writing the equation in logarithmic form.

$$\log(P_2) = \log(1) + 1.41 \log(2)$$
$$\log(1) = 0$$
$$1.41 \log(2) = 1.41 \times 0.301 = 0.4244$$
$$\log(P_2) = 0.4244$$
$$P_2 = \text{antilog}\ (0.4244)$$
$$P_2 = 2.657 \text{ atmospheres}$$

The compressed gas reached a pressure of 2.66 atmospheres when its volume was halved adiabatically. If the process had been isothermal then Boyle's law would have yielded

$$P_2 = P_1 \left(\frac{V_1}{V_2}\right),$$

and

$$P_2 = 2 \text{ atmospheres.}$$

The extra pressure generated in an adiabatic compression came from the work done on the gas to increase its temperature.

PROBLEM 6

(a) Expired gas volumes measured by spirometry and gas meters are at ambient temperature, T_A, and barometric pressure, P_B, and saturated with water vapour, so that a partial pressure of water, P_{H_2O} exists in the expired gas. Develop a formula to convert these A.T.P.S. (ambient temperature and pressure, saturated) volumes to standard conditions of 0°C and 760 mm Hg, dry (S.T.P.D.).

(b) A ventilator is to be tested on a compliance made from a large glass bottle. A volume cycled ventilator is set to deliver a tidal volume of 500 ml. The volume of the air in the bottle and ventilator connections is 60 litres at 1033 cm H_2O pressure (1 atmosphere), and the 500 ml is added to this volume during inspiration. The process may be assumed equivalent to the compression of 60 litres to 59.5 litres. What is the compliance of this system if the compression is assumed to be adiabatic? If isothermal? Express compliance in ml/cm H_2O.

Chapter 7

VAPOURS

THE BOUNDARY BETWEEN THE LIQUID AND GASEOUS STATES

As a gas is cooled, the K.E. of its molecules declines until intermolecular binding forces begin to be significant. At the same time the volume of the gas shrinks, bringing the gas molecules closer together so that they begin to interfere with each other's movements. The gas begins to deviate from its ideal behaviour, and the ideal gas law and other laws based upon it may not apply accurately. Finally, as the temperature is reduced further, the intermolecular binding forces become sufficiently strong to constitute a liquid.

Compression can also be used to liquify a gas. The gas molecules can be forced so closely together that they function as a liquid, but only if the temperature is below a critical value for each kind of gas. Above the *critical temperature,* the gas molecules are so energetic that, close packing notwithstanding, the low energy bonds between molecules which constitute a liquid are still insignificant when compared with the K.E. of the molecules. Table XII lists the critical temperatures of gases used in anaesthetic practice.

Nitrous oxide, carbon dioxide and cyclopropane are gases whose critical temperatures are above room temperature (20°C), and so these gases are in the liquid state in full cylinders at room temperature. Oxygen, however, has a critical temperature well below room temperature, and so it is not in the liquid state in cylinders at room temperature, no matter how high the cylinder pressure. Ether and halothane and the other liquid anaesthetics, on the other hand, have critical temperatures so much higher than room temperature that they are liquids at a pressure of one atmosphere.

We usually employ the term *vapour* to refer to the gaseous

TABLE XII

CRITICAL TEMPERATURES (K)*

Air	132.7
Nitrogen (N_2)	126.0
Oxygen (O_2)	154.576
Carbon dioxide	304.0
Nitrous oxide	309.5
Helium	5.07
Xenon	289.6
Water	647
Ethyl chloride	460.2
Ethylene	282.9
Cyclopropane	397.7

* R. C. Weast (Ed.): *Handbook of Chemistry and Physics*. Chemical Rubber Company Press, Cleveland, Ohio, U.S.A.

form of a substance which is normally a liquid. However, a more rigorous definition would read: a vapour is a substance in its gaseous state but below its critical temperature. Using this definition, cyclopropane, nitrous oxide and carbon dioxide are all vapours at room temperature.

ISOTHERMS

The relations between pressure, volume and temperature, for a substance which exists as a vapour, are usually plotted as *isotherms* on a graph of pressure against volume. Each isotherm traces the relation between pressure and volume at one particular temperature. Figure 40 shows typical isotherms, with the critical temperature isotherm distinguishable as a heavier line.

At temperatures far above the critical temperature, the isotherms become rectangular hyperbolas; the gas behaviour is ideal, and Boyle's law holds. The equation for the isotherms has the form $P = 1/V$, the form that was plotted and named in Problem 1.

At temperatures below the critical temperature, the substance may exist as a vapour, or as a liquid, or as a mixture of both, depending upon its volume and pressure. The isotherms become horizontal as the vapour condenses into a liquid because a decrease in volume does not raise the pressure, but instead converts more vapour into liquid. Only when the volume has decreased

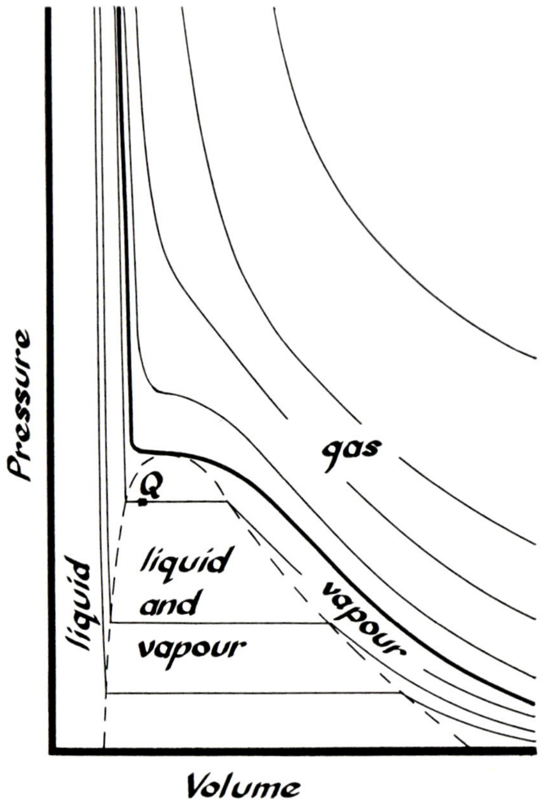

Figure 40. Isotherms.

sufficiently to convert all of the vapour into liquid does the pressure rise. The area of Figure 40 containing the horizontal portions of the isotherms is outlined by a dashed line. It encloses an area of the diagram where vapour and liquid exist in equilibrium with each other. To the left of the liquid-vapour area, and below the critical isotherm, the substance is liquid. The isotherms rise steeply indicating that very large pressures are generated when a liquid is compressed; liquids are therefore said to be incompressible. To the right of the liquid-vapour area, and below the critical isotherm, the substance is a vapour, and the ideal gas law may be used to approximate the behaviour of the vapour.

To illustrate the use of isotherms, we can trace the pressure-volume relationship in a nitrous oxide cylinder as it empties isothermally at a room temperature of 20°C. (The process is isothermal if the cylinder is emptied over a long period of time.) Since the critical temperature for nitrous oxide is 36.5°C from Table XII, the isotherm for 20°C lies below the critical isotherm, and the contents of a full cylinder of nitrous oxide might be at a point Q in Figure 40.

The withdrawal of gas from a cylinder is equivalent to increasing the volume occupied by the gas left inside; that is, a decrease in the amount of gas in a fixed volume may be thought of as equivalent to an increase in the volume of the same amount. Therefore, we can follow the changes in pressure as the cylinder empties by moving along the isotherm for 20°C from point Q towards increasing volume.

At first, the full cylinder contains both liquid and vapour, and as gas is withdrawn pressure stays constant until all the liquid has become vapour (the horizontal portion of the isotherm). At that point the cylinder contains only vapour, and the pressure declines gradually as the cylinder empties (the curved, right-hand portion of the isotherm).

We conclude from the nitrous oxide example that for gases below their critical temperature, and existing in liquid form in cylinders, the cylinder pressure is not proportional to the amount of gas in the cylinder. The only way to determine the amount of gas in a cylinder containing a partially liquified gas is to weigh the cylinder and compare it with the empty weight.

For gases above their critical temperatures, like oxygen (>−118°C) or nitrous oxide (>36.5°C), the cylinders contain only gas, and the cylinder pressure is therefore proportional to the amount of gas in the cylinder.

THE VAPOUR PRESSURE CURVE

In the previous section we defined a vapour as a gas that was at a temperature below its critical temperature. Figure 40 showed that, at temperatures below the critical temperature, a substance can be a vapour, a liquid or a mixture of both. The horizontal portions of the isotherms (enclosed by a dashed line) mark the region where the liquid and vapour are in equilibrium. At this equilibrium point, the vapour is termed a *saturated vapour*, and the pressure (for any given temperature) is called the *vapour pressure* or *saturated vapour pressure* at that temperature. If we plot pressure versus the temperatures for the horizontal portions of the isotherms in Figure 40, then we obtain a graph of vapour pressures against their corresponding temperatures which is called a *vapour pressure curve*. Figure 41 shows vapour pressure curves for some volatile anaesthetics.

From Figure 41 we can read the vapour pressure of an anaesthetic for any given temperature. If these temperature and pressure conditions prevail, then the liquid and vapour forms of the anaesthetic are in equilibrium. If the temperature rises then the

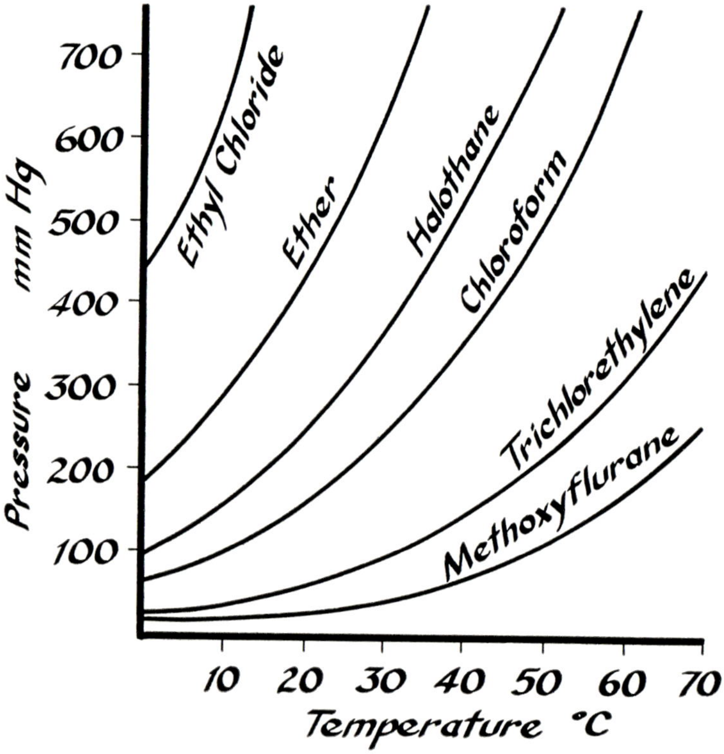

Figure 41. Vapour pressure curves for some volatile anaesthetics.

equilibrium is unbalanced, and more liquid evaporates until the vapour pressure has increased to a new equilibrium point. The latent heat of vaporization is supplied by the same energy source that increased the temperature. Similarly, if energy is extracted, the temperature falls, and vapour condenses until the vapour pressure has fallen to a new equilibrium pressure.

Figure 41 may also be used to predict what happens when partial pressure changes occur. Consider a sealed container containing only anaesthetic. At any given temperature the liquid and vapour will be in equilibrium at the vapour pressure. Now, if the container is opened, then the vapour dissipates into the open air. The partial pressure of the anaesthetic is very much lower than its vapour pressure so that the equilibrium is far off balance, and the liquid anaesthetic evaporates in a futile attempt to establish a partial pressure in the atmosphere equal to the vapour pressure. The latent heat is drawn from the body of the liquid and its surroundings causing a local drop in temperature.

When an open container of halothane is maintained at 50°C by a supply of energy, the liquid anaesthetic evaporates in an attempt to establish an equilibrium with its vapour at a vapour pressure of 760 mm Hg (that is, equal to standard atmospheric pressure). Therefore, bubbles of pure halothane vapour (whose internal pressure is equal to the vapour pressure) are not crushed by atmospheric pressure as they would be if their internal pressure was below 760 mm Hg; the halothane is boiling. Another definition of boiling point is thus, the temperature at which the vapour pressure of a substance is equal to the external pressure (usually standardized at one atmosphere pressure).

HUMIDITY

Atmospheric air is a mixture of gases and water vapour. Table XIII lists points on the vapour pressure curve for water, and thereby indicates the highest partial pressure of water (P_{H_2O}) which may exist in air at any given temperature. Air that contains water vapour at a partial pressure equal to the vapour pressure at that temperature is said to be fully saturated. If the air is then cooled, then the equilibrium shifts to convert water

TABLE XIII

VAPOUR PRESSURE OF WATER*

Temperature °C	*Vapour Pressure mm Hg*
0	4.579
5	6.543
10	9.209
15	12.788
20	17.535
25	23.756
30	31.824
35	42.175
37	47.067
40	55.324
45	71.88
50	92.51
55	118.04
60	149.38
65	187.54
70	233.7
75	289.1
80	355.1
85	433.6
90	525.76
95	633.90
100	760.00

* R. C. Weast (Ed.): *Handbook of Chemistry and Physics,* 54th Edition. Chemical Rubber Company Press, Cleveland, Ohio, U.S.A., 1973-1974.

vapour to liquid water; water condenses on the cooling surfaces that remove the latent heat of vaporization.

For example, when air saturated with water vapour is expired, it rapidly cools to room temperature (20°C). P_{H_2O} must fall from the vapour pressure at 37°C, 47 mm Hg, to the vapour pressure at 20°C, 20 mm Hg. The excess water vapour condenses to liquid on surfaces that conduct away the latent heat of vaporization (metals are good heat conductors).

The water vapour content of air may be expressed as a relative humidity or as an absolute humidity. *Absolute humidity* is defined as the mass of water vapour per unit volume, while *relative humidity* is expressed as a percentage of the vapour pressure, that is

$$\text{relative humidity } (\%) = 100 \times \frac{P_{H_2O}}{\begin{array}{c}\text{vapour pressure}\\ \text{(at the same temperature)}\end{array}}.$$

The meaning of the terms relative and absolute humidity are perhaps best explained by an example showing their calculation.

Given a temperature of 20°C, and a P_{H_2O} of 10 mm Hg, what is the relative and absolute humidity? From Table XIII, the vapour pressure of water at 20°C is 17.5 mm Hg, and so

$$\text{relative humidity} = 100 \times \frac{10 \text{ mm Hg}}{17.5 \text{ mm Hg}} = 57\%.$$

To calculate the absolute humidity we must calculate the mass of water vapour present per unit volume. Recalling that Dalton's law says that the P_{H_2O} is the pressure that the water vapour alone would exert in a volume V at 20°C, we can use the ideal gas law to determine the mass of water present.

$$P_{H_2O} \cdot V = nRT,$$

and

$$\frac{n}{V} = \frac{P_{H_2O}}{RT}.$$

We know that:

$$R = 62 \text{ mm Hg} \cdot \text{l/mol} \cdot \text{K},$$

$$T = 20°\text{C} = 293 \text{ K},$$

and

$$P = 10 \text{ mm Hg}.$$

Therefore,

$$\frac{n}{V} = \frac{10 \text{ mm Hg} \cdot \text{mol} \cdot \text{K}}{62 \text{ mm Hg} \cdot \text{l} \cdot 293 \text{ K}} = 5.5 \times 10^{-4} \frac{\text{mol}}{\text{l}}.$$

Since the molecular weight of water is 18 g/mol;

$$\text{absolute humidity} = 5.5 \times 10^{-4} \frac{\text{mol}}{\text{l}} \times 18 \frac{\text{g}}{\text{mol}},$$

$$\text{absolute humidity} = 9.9 \times 10^{-3} \text{ g/l (or kg/kl or kg/m}^3\text{)},$$

$$\text{or, absolute humidity} = 9.9 \text{ mg/litre (or g/kl or g/m}^3\text{)}.$$

The calculation above assumed that the absolute humidity of air saturated with water vapour at 20°C was unknown. However, if the absolute humidity of 17.3×10^{-3} g/l corresponding to 100 percent relative humidity had been known, then, knowing the relative humidity as 57 percent,

$$\text{absolute humidity} = 17.3 \times 10^{-3} \frac{\text{g}}{\text{l}} \times \frac{57}{100},$$

$$\text{absolute humidity} = 9.9 \times 10^{-3} \text{ g/l}.$$

Relative humidity may be measured most accurately by determining the temperature of the *dew point.* This is the point at which a polished metal container is cooled just enough so that its surface becomes cloudy with condensed water droplets. Suppose, for example, that room air at 20°C is found to have a dew point temperature of 10°C. At 10°C water begins condensing out of the air which means that the air is saturated at 10°C. The vapour pressure at 10°C (from Table XIII) is 9.2 mm Hg, and this is the partial pressure of the water vapour in the room air at 20°C. Relative humidity is therefore,

$$\frac{9.2}{17.5} \times 100 = 52.6\%.$$

A simpler way to measure relative humidity is to use wet- and dry-bulb thermometers. Two thermometers are placed side by side with the bulb of one kept moist by a wick dipped in water. Because the water evaporates in an attempt to saturate the air, it draws the latent heat of vaporization from its surroundings thereby lowering the temperature of the wet-bulb thermometer. The lower the relative humidity, the more water tends to evaporate, so that the difference in temperature between wet- and dry-bulb thermometers increases. Tables provide a listing of relative humidity versus wet- and dry-bulb thermometer readings.

HUMIDIFIERS

When the humidification of the nasopharynx has been bypassed with an endotracheal tube or a tracheostomy, the inspired gases require artificial humidification. Normally, alveolar air is fully saturated with water vapour at 37°C; a relative humidity of 100 percent, and an absolute humidity of 44×10^{-3} kg/m³ (g/l). Humidification of the inspired gases can be achieved in three ways; a condenser in the breathing circuit at the point of connection with the patient, the addition of water vapour to the inspired gas by passing it over or through heated water, and the addition of an aerosol of microdroplets of water to the inspired gas.

The condenser humidifier is made up of a number of wire gauzes or a series of parallel small bore tubes enclosed within a larger tube through which the respired air passes. The large surface area of the wire gauzes, or small tubes, acts to condense the water vapour from the saturated expired gas and is warmed in the process. During inspiration, the condenser yields its heat and moisture to the inspired gas. The dead space and flow resistance of the condenser can be made acceptably small, but the large surface area tends to collect secretions, increasing the resistance and the possibility of bacterial colonization. The condenser humidifier performs best when the inspired gas is cool and partly humidified but fails when dry gases from cylinders or piped supplies are used. The condenser humidifier's disadvantages have caused its failure in clinical practice.

The hot water humidifier consists of a water reservoir through which the inspired gas is bubbled. The water is heated by a thermostatically controlled element to provide the necessary heat of vaporization, and the gas is bubbled through the hot water so as to obtain a gas-water interface with a large surface area. The hot water humidifier is quite adequate in its ability to provide saturated gas at 37°C at the humidifier outlet, but because of the low specific heat of gases, the delivery tube temperature falls very quickly to room temperature with a consequent loss of water vapour by condensation. This problem, however, can be overcome by placing the thermostat sensor close to the patient end of the delivery tube and insulating and warming the delivery tube.

Aerosol humidifiers add microdroplet aerosols of water to the inspired gas. The aerosols may be produced by ultrasonic nebulizers, gas driven nebulizers utilizing the venturi effect and mechanical nebulizers like the spinning disc. In this way, a water-gas interface of large surface area can be produced to aid vaporization, but the heat of vaporization must be supplied from the surrounding air or by heating the water. The lifetime of the microdroplets depends upon their size, the relative humidity of the surrounding gas, the temperature, and the microdroplet per volume density. If conditions are such that the mist exists for long enough to be inspired, then the microdroplets are deposited throughout the airway, depending upon their size. The water content of a volume of air containing an aerosol may exceed that of saturation, but this is because the water is partially in liquid form as microdroplets rather than in vapour form. As yet, it is not clear whether the water content of inspired air should be liquid (microdroplet) or vapour.

ANAESTHETIC VAPORIZERS

The characteristics of volatile anaesthetics which determine the operation of an anaesthetic vaporizer are listed in Table XIV. The vapour pressure at 20°C indicates how far away from a liquid-vapour equilibrium the anaesthetic will be in an open container and is therefore a measure of its tendency to vaporize. The amount of heat required for vaporization to proceed is given by the latent heat of vaporization for each anaesthetic. Ease of vaporization is therefore associated with a high vapour pressure and a low latent heat of vaporization. The range of concentrations used in anaesthesia determines the concentration

TABLE XIV

CHARACTERISTICS OF VOLATILE ANAESTHETICS

Anaesthetic	*Range of Concentration (Vol. %) Used in Anaesthesia*	*Boiling Point °C @ 760 mm Hg*[1]	*Vapour Pressure mm Hg @ 20°C*[2]	*Saturation Concentration (Vol. %) @ 20°C*	*Latent Heat of Vaporization @ 20°C cal./g*[2]
Diethyl ether	3.5-4.5	34.6	442	58	94.4
Chloroform	1.5	61.5	160	19.7	59.0
Trichloroethylene	2-7.5	86.7	64.5	7.5	57.0
Halothane	1-3	50.2	243.3	31.7	37.0
Methoxyflurane	1-2	105	23	3.03	59.5

[1] Paul G. Stecker (Ed.): *The Merck Index*. Merck and Company Ltd., Rahway, New Jersey, U.S.A.

[2] Secher, O.: Physical and chemical data on anaesthetics. *Acta Anaesthesiologica Scandinavica*, Supplementum XLII, 1971.

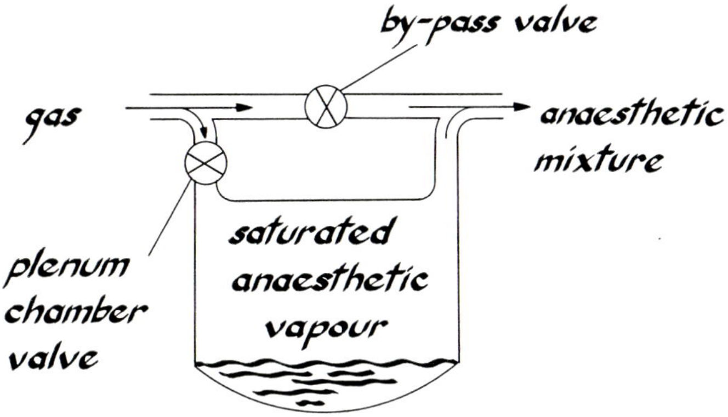

Figure 42. Simple plenum vaporizer.

of the anaesthetic vapour which will be produced by the vaporizer. Since this concentration is well below the saturation concentration of the volatile anaesthetics, the vaporizer need not saturate the inspired gas passing through it, and, in fact, most vaporizers incorporate a by-pass valve (Figure 42) so that the flow from the vaporizing chamber can be diluted with fresh gas.

Most anaesthetic vaporizers are based upon the simple plenum vaporizer pictured in Figure 42. The term plenum, originally used in physics to describe a space full of matter, was later adapted to describe the ventilation of a building by a forced inflow of fresh air which expelled the stale air and hence, is used to describe a vaporizer in which fresh gas is forced into the vaporizing chamber thereby expelling the gas and vapour mixture.

Ideally, the plenum vaporizer operates by diluting the gas from the vaporizing chamber which is saturated with anaesthetic vapour, with fresh gas via the by-pass valve; all at a constant temperature. With a known saturation concentration at room temperature for each anaesthetic, the ratio of by-pass flow to vaporizing chamber flow may be calculated so as to produce any desired anaesthetic concentration. Unfortunately, such a situation is ideal rather than practical, since it depends upon the ability of the vaporizing chamber to supply any set flow at the saturation concentration.

The design of a vaporizing chamber to provide the conversion of liquid anaesthetic to vapour at a constant temperature and independent of flow depends upon two main factors; the surface area of the liquid-gas interface, and the supply of heat for the latent heat of vaporization. The first factor is not troublesome. For example, in the Boyle bottle and Copper Kettle vaporizers, surface area is made sufficiently large by bubbling the gas through the liquid anaesthetic. Another method is to use a system of wicks, such as those employed in the Fluotec vaporizers.

The second factor, the heat supply, is difficult to manage. Consider what happens in a plenum vaporizer when it is turned on (Figure 43). Initially, the chamber/by-pass flow ratio is set to supply the desired concentration of anaesthetic vapour from the vaporizer. However, if the walls of the vaporizing chamber do not conduct heat well, nor store heat, then the temperature of the liquid anaesthetic and the vaporizing chamber falls as the heat is used to supply the latent heat of vaporization. The rate of vaporization slows, and the vapour concentration falls. As the liquid temperature falls, heat flow into the chamber increases due to the temperature gradient. The anaesthetist now increases the chamber/by-pass flow ratio so as to maintain the anaesthetic concentration and causes the same changes all over again. Eventually an equilibrium is reached where the temperature inside the chamber is low enough to cause a heat flow sufficient to vaporize enough liquid anaesthetic for an increased chamber gas flow necessitated by the decrease in the saturation concentration with temperature. The start and equilibrium conditions in a plenum vaporizer are shown in Figure 43.

The characteristics of each anaesthetic given in Table XIV will determine how extreme these heat problems will be in the vaporizer. For example, it is apparent that the vaporizing chamber for ether, which requires 94.4 calories to vaporize one gram, will reach a lower temperature than the vaporizing chamber for halothane, which requires only 37 calories. Exacerbating this temperature difference is the fact that ether is less potent than halothane, and so more ether must be vaporized than halothane. However, ether's saving feature is its high vapour pressure and

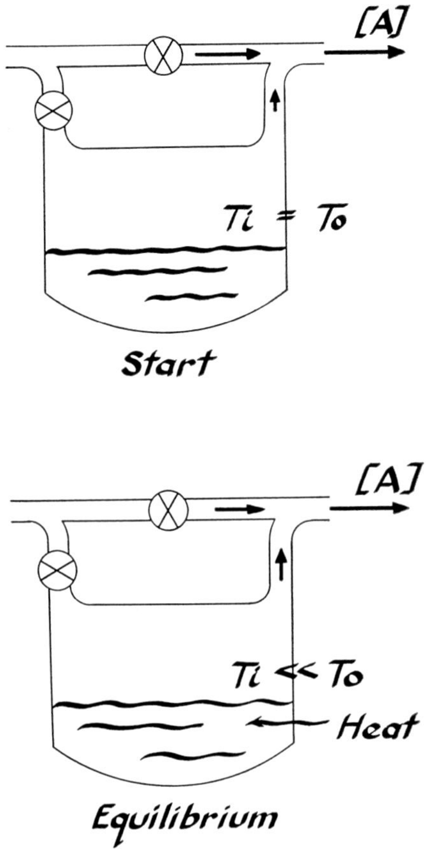

Figure 43. Initial and equilibrium conditions for a plenum vaporizer.

saturation concentration, almost double that of halothane, which makes it possible to vaporize enough ether in a vaporizer like the Boyle bottle with its glass-walled vaporizing chamber which conducts heat very poorly. The Boyle bottle nevertheless requires manual adjustment to compensate for changes in anaesthetic vapour concentration with temperature and produces a surge of vapour when first turned on and when shaken.

In order to produce a calibrated vaporizer which produces a known anaesthetic concentration over a range of gas flows, some method of supplying heat and compensating for temperature changes must be incorporated into vaporizers. Since the supply of the latent heat of vaporization comes from the walls of the vaporizing chamber and its surroundings, the chamber walls are usually made of copper; a good conductor of heat and (because of a high specific heat) a good reservoir of heat. The Copper Kettle, for example, is made of copper and also fixed to a copper plate on the anaesthetic machine. By these means the temperature drop in the vaporizing chamber is minimized.

The changes in the chamber/by-pass flow ratio required to maintain a constant output vapour concentration in the face of temperature changes may be done by automatic compensation or by the anaesthetist. In the case of the Drager Vapor vaporizer, the vaporizing chamber temperature is read from a built-in thermometer, and the anaesthetist changes the flow valves according to a compensation chart. Alternatively, in the Fluotec vaporizers, the adjustment is automated through the use of temperature sensitive valves.

The plenum vaporizers described so far are used in systems which supply the inlet gas under sufficient pressure to produce the necessary flow through the vaporizer, and their flow resistance is, therefore, too high for use as draw-over vaporizers where the flow is produced by the effort of the patient. Draw-over vaporizers are thus, low flow resistance vaporizers. Because the flow is intermittent in draw-over vaporizers, their requirements for temperature control or compensation are even more rigorous than in plenum vaporizers (steady flows) unless the calibration is restricted to a particular range of intermittent flows.

One other method of producing a known anaesthetic concentration is the injection or drip-feed vaporizer. In this simple device liquid anaesthetic is continually dripped, or injected at regular intervals, into the stream of ventilating gas. The flow of anaesthetic required to produce a particular concentration may be calculated (assuming complete vaporization) from first principles by vaporizing the required mass of anaesthetic into the known volume.

Vaporizers can be used in hyperbaric or hypobaric pressure environments with little change in their clinical operation because the vapour pressure curve is independent of ambient pressure and depends only upon ambient temperature. The partial pressure of anaesthetic produced by a vaporizer, therefore, remains practically independent of ambient pressure. Since the partial pressure remains the same, the concentration will vary inversely with ambient pressure, but because the density of the vapour varies directly with ambient pressure, the mass flow of anaesthetic remains the same at all ambient pressures, dependent only upon ambient temperature.

PROBLEM 7

Calculate:

(a) The flow of liquid halothane in a drip or injection feed vaporizer to produce a concentration of 1% halothane (volume/volume) in a 6 litre per minute flow (gas and vapour).

(b) The flow of saturated vapour (at room temperature) from the vaporizing chamber of a plenum vaporizer for the same 6 litre/min. flow of 1% halothane anaesthesia.

(c) The electrical power (watts) of a heater to keep the chamber of the plenum vaporizer at room temperature.

(d) The volume of liquid halothane vaporized in the plenum vaporizer in one hour.

Useful information:

Halothane; molecular weight = 197
liquid density = 1.86 g/ml,
latent heat of vaporization = 37 cal./g,
boiling point at 760 mm Hg = 50°C,
thermal capacity = 0.19 cal./g/°C,
vapour pressure at 20°C = 241 mm Hg.
Barometric pressure = 760 mm Hg.
Room temperature = 20°C.

Chapter 8

FLUIDS

DEFINITION

AT THE MOLECULAR LEVEL a liquid differs from a solid in that the bonds holding the molecules together are weak and fleeting, whereas the bonds in a solid are strong enough to hold the molecules in a rigid lattice structure. Liquid molecules are free to wander throughout the bulk of the liquid, and it is this property of molecular freedom that characterizes a liquid.

Consider a steel bar twisted in opposite directions at each end. For a certain amount of shearing force (stress) applied, the bar will deform (strain) elastically to a corresponding angle, and at that point the internal and external forces will reach an equilibrium. No further movement results; the system of forces is static, sustaining a fixed shear stress and resulting shear strain indefinitely. Contrast this behaviour with that of a liquid like water. Water cannot even withstand the shear stress applied by gravity, and it deforms (the layers of water slide past each other) until it takes the shape of its container. The smallest of shear forces applied to a liquid will produce an infinite strain; in other words, the liquid deforms until the shear force is relieved. This example leads us to the engineering definition of a fluid: A *fluid* is a substance that cannot sustain shear forces. A

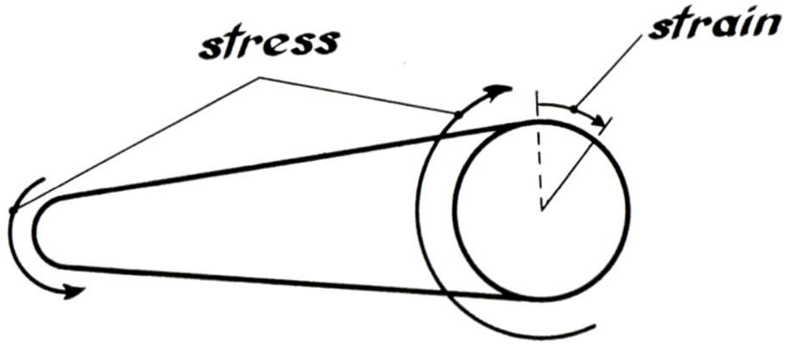

Figure 44. Stress and strain in a twisted rod.

similar argument can also be applied to gases, and so the term fluid includes both gases and liquids.

Rigorously, the definition of a fluid is only true of the static situation where no fluid movement occurs. Under dynamic conditions, during fluid movement when the layers of fluid are sliding past each other, the fluid does sustain small shear forces between the layers. For example, thick tar is a fluid that will hold the shape of a bar. When the bar is twisted in the same way as the steel bar, the tar appears to sustain the applied shear stress, but upon close inspection it can be seen that the tar is shearing, albeit slowly. Eventually, the tar will deform enough to relieve the shear stress. The shear forces are only sustained by the tar during the time that the strain is increasing.

Another example of shear stress sustained by a fluid in the dynamic situation but not the static is that of the action of a fan blade cutting through air, and thereby deforming the fluid air. At very low speeds of rotation the air is deformed with very little force applied to the fan blade, but at high speeds the force required is large. In other words, the fluid air only sustains noticeable shear stress when the rate of change of strain with time is high. The property of fluids which gives rise to these dynamic shear stresses is called viscosity and will be considered in the next chapter on fluid flow.

SURFACE TENSION

Fluids are commonly divided into the two subclasses, liquids and gases, because of their differing characteristics. A liquid occupies a definite volume and can, therefore, have a free surface, but a gas expands to fill any volume in which it is placed, and so has no free surface. A gas is compressible by moderate pressure, but a liquid is only slightly compressed by very high pressures and so is considered incompressible.

The free surface of a liquid, shown in Figure 45(a), is composed of molecules which are attracted to their neighbours in all directions except that away from the surface. These forces of attraction are the low energy bonds that make the fluid a liquid rather than a gas. They pull at the surface molecules, continually attempting to shrink the surface, and produce the effect of

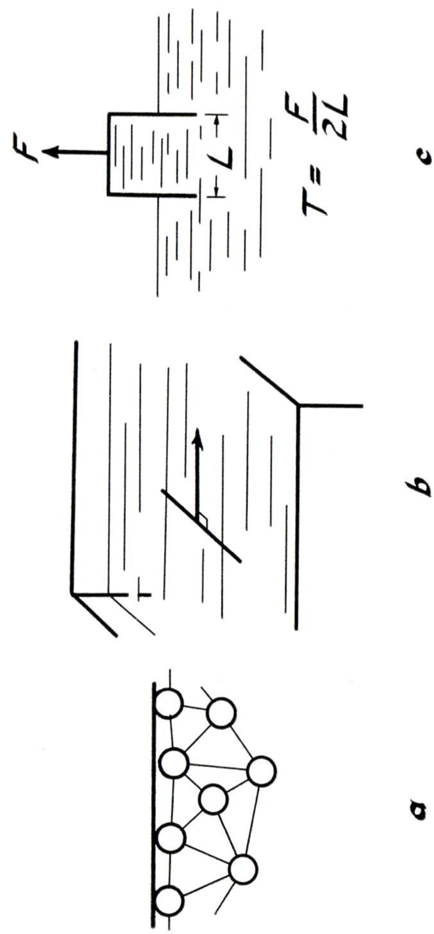

Figure 45. Definition of surface tension.

surface tension. Outside a gravitational field, liquid surrounded by free space or gas adopts a spherical configuration because this geometric form has the smallest surface area.

Figure 45(b) demonstrates the definition of *surface tension* as the force of contraction across a line in the liquid surface. Both the force and the line lie in the plane of the liquid surface and are mutually perpendicular. Surface tension is measured (Figure 45(c)) by dipping a wire frame into the particular liquid and measuring the force at which the frame breaks away from the surface. This force divided by twice the length of the wire frame is equal to the surface tension. The S.I. unit of surface tension is thus the newton per metre, abbreviated N/m. As an example, the surface tension of water at 20°C is 75 mN/m (millinewtons per metre).

An important application of the surface tension concept for anaesthetists involves the surface tension of the fluid lining the alveoli of the lungs. Since the alveoli may be approximated by fluid lined spheres or bubbles, they would be expected to obey *Laplace's law* (Pierre Simon, Marquis de Laplace, 1749-1827, French mathematician and astronomer), that is $P \propto \frac{2T}{r}$, where:

P = the pressure inside a bubble,
T = the surface tension of the liquid comprising the bubble,
r = the radius of the bubble.

Laplace's law says that the surface tension in a bubble tends to shrink the surface area and so cause a build-up of pressure within the bubble; the larger the bubble, the smaller the pressure. Since the alveoli of the lungs may be considered to be a group of interconnected bubbles, we would therefore expect that small alveoli would be more difficult to expand than large alveoli, and that small alveoli would tend to empty into larger alveoli. This situation would be detrimental to the lungs and does not usually happen because of the presence of a surface active substance (surfactant) in the fluid lining the alveoli. The surfactant molecules interpose themselves between the liquid molecules and reduce the surface tension by replacing the large liquid-liquid attraction forces by the smaller liquid-surfactant attraction. The surfactant mechanism also has the property of increasing the amount of surfactant on the interior surface as the alveolus shrinks. Therefore, although Laplace's Law does apply to the alveolus, its consequences are nullified by the alteration in surface tension due to the presence of surfactant.

FLUID STATICS

A fluid in *static equilibrium* is one in which there are no shear forces present; one fluid layer does not slide relative to the next. The only forces that can act upon a fluid in static equilibrium are compressive forces. *Pascal's* important *law* of fluid behaviour states that the pressure in a static fluid is the same in all directions.

Suppose that we squeeze a fluid by compressing it in a piston and cylinder arrangement. If the weight of the fluid is negligible, then the pressure throughout the fluid is the same. In other words, the sides of the cylinder, and the top and bottom, all have the same force per unit area exerted on them as is being ex-

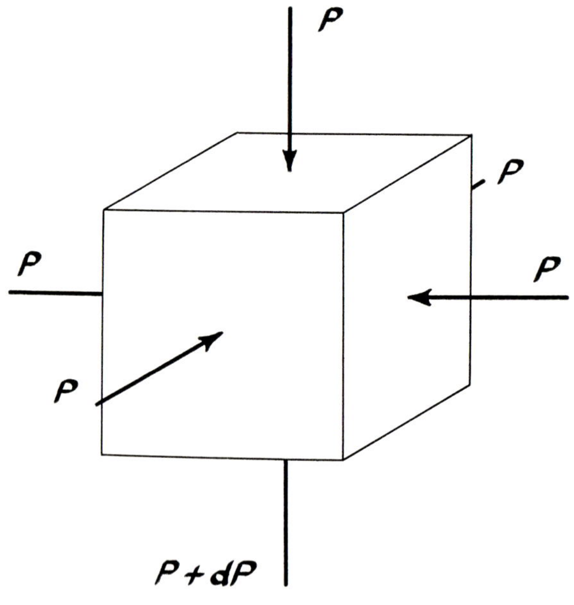

Figure 46. Illustration of Pascal's law.

erted by the piston. The forces on a small object in the fluid are compressive; the same from all directions at once, and also the same no matter where the object is located in the fluid.

Contrast this behaviour with that of a solid under the same conditions. The force of a piston on a solid only acts in the direction of the piston movement, and so only the bottom of the cylinder would be subjected to a pressure. A small object embedded in the solid would also be subjected to forces only in the direction of piston movement.

Now consider a fluid in static equilibrium acted upon only by the force of gravity. Figure 46 shows an elemental cube of fluid within the fluid bulk, with pressures on each of its faces. The pressure on the bottom face is higher than that on the top face by an amount dependent upon the weight of the cube. The pressures on the side faces are equal and opposite in direction to each other since the cube is in static equilibrium. Let the pressure on the top face be P and that on the bottom face be $P + dP$. The weight of the cube is

$$\rho \cdot G \cdot dh \cdot dA,$$

where:

ρ = the density of the fluid,
G = the acceleration due to gravity,
dh = the height of the elemental cube,
dA = the cross-sectional area of the elemental cube.

Since the cube is in static equilibrium, the weight of the cube must equal the increase in the force on the bottom plate, and therefore

$$-dA \cdot dP = \rho \cdot G \cdot dh \cdot dA,$$

and

$$-dP = \rho \cdot G \cdot dh.$$

The negative sign indicates that the forces are acting in opposite directions. The differential equation above is a fundamental relation in fluid statics, and states that the pressure in a fluid increases with both depth and fluid density.

The equation describes the conditions in a manometer, a device which measures pressure by balancing the pressure to be measured against the pressure developed at the bottom of a column of fluid in static equilibrium. Liquids are used as the fluid in manometers because of their high density and incompressibility. Liquid densities can be considered constant, and integration of the fluid statics equation yields,

$$\int - dP = \int \rho G dh,$$
$$-\int dP = \rho G \int dh,$$
$$P = \rho GH,$$

and

where:

> P is the pressure exerted at the bottom of the manometer,
> ρ is the density of the liquid used in the manometer,
> G is the acceleration due to gravity,

and

> H is the height of the manometer column.

Note that because ρ is constant, the fluid statics equation integrates to a linear relationship between pressure and column height. If ρ was a function of height as it is in the atmosphere (because air is compressible), then the integration is more complicated, and the resulting relation between P and H is nonlinear.

The manometer equation above can be used to determine the pressure *(P)* due to any differences in liquid levels *(H)*. It can be applied to situations where two or more liquids (not mixed) comprise the total difference in height between levels by adding the pressures resulting from the application of the manometer equation to each liquid in turn. In medicine, where the use of manometers to measure pressure was widespread, pressure was expressed as manometer column heights, in units such as mm Hg and cm H_2O, so as to avoid the calculation of pressure using the manometer equation, and this practice is still used.

SOLUBILITY

Anaesthetists use fluids which are mostly in the form of solutions. The term *solution* is difficult to define rigorously, but it could be described as a fluid consisting of more than one kind of molecule and uniformly intermingled. Ideally the constituent molecules of a solution are completely indifferent to each other, and in this respect, the gas mixtures used in anaesthesia are almost ideal solutions. However, many solutions are made from constituents that do interact with each other; either physically, such as in the case of polarized water molecules clustering around ions; or chemically, such as the chemical reaction of carbon dioxide and water. Such solutions, although not ideal in behaviour, may still be treated as such under limited conditions.

The best way of describing the properties of solutions, like solubility and diffusion, is by using current theories of thermodynamics, thereby providing a generalized description which may be applied to any given situation. However, since anaesthetists are not trained in this field and such training is outside the scope of this book, the descriptions in this chapter are conventional and treat specific situations. Generalizations are therefore difficult to make.

A solution is said to be saturated when an equilibrium is established between the two processes of *solute* molecules (those in the minority) going into and coming out of solution in the *solvent* (the substance with the majority of molecules). The concentration (mass/mass) of the solution at saturation is a measure of the ability of the solute to dissolve in a particular solvent and is called the *solubility*. Solubility is affected by temperature, and in the case of solutions of gases in liquids, it is affected by pressure. Solutions of solids in liquids show a solubility which increases with temperature, but the reverse is true for solutions of gases in liquids. This contrasting behaviour occurs because the lattice structure of solids breaks more easily at higher temperatures, whereas the increased K.E. of gas molecules at high temperatures tends to keep them in the gaseous state.

The anaesthetist is primarily concerned with solutions of gases in liquids because the solubility of the anaesthetic gases and vapours in blood and tissues largely determines the pharmacokinetics of their induction and recovery; agents with high solubility are slower than low solubility agents because more (mass) of the anaesthetic must be transferred in order to reach a given concentration. In addition to temperature, the solubility of gases in liquids (the mass of gas per unit volume of liquid) is also affected by the pressure of the gaseous phase. Consider a single gas confined with a single liquid, and allowed to reach equilibrium. At equilibrium there will be a liquid phase, a solution of gas molecules in the liquid; and a gaseous phase, a solution of liquid molecules (in the gaseous state) in the gas. At equilibrium, the concentration of the gas in the liquid solution corresponds to the partial pressure of the gas in the gaseous phase. The anaesthetist usually refers to the equilibrium concentration of the gas in the liquid phase in terms of its partial pressure in the gaseous phase. The solubility of the gas in the liquid depends directly upon the partial pressure of the gas phase, that is

$$\frac{n_L}{V_L} \propto P,$$

where:

n_L = the number of moles of dissolved gas,
V_L = the volume of liquid solution,
P = the partial pressure of the gas phase.
n_L/V_L = the concentration of the gas in the liquid phase ≡ solubility.

Here we have expressed concentration in moles per unit volume, but mass per unit volume or mass per mass or moles per moles could have been used as well.

William Henry (1775-1836), the English chemist, investigated the above relation and found that it was linear for ideal gases that formed ideal solutions; in other words, for gases that are far above their critical temperatures and pressures and that do not interact with the liquid molecules. Anaesthetists, however, are interested in liquid solutions of anaesthetic vapours which are below their critical temperatures and in respiratory gases, such as carbon dioxide, which interact with water. Despite these departures from the ideal, the linear relationship between concentration and partial pressure stated by Henry is accurate enough for most anaesthetic situations, but each situation should be carefully examined for deviations from the ideal behaviour.

Henry's law states that,

$$\frac{n_L}{V_L} = K_T P,$$

where K_T is the constant of proportionality (the slope of the concentration versus partial pressure graph) at temperature T and is called the *solubility coefficient.* A dimensional analysis shows that K_T is measured in units of concentration per pressure, such as moles per litre per mm Hg. The solubility coefficient is not actually a constant for any particular gas and liquid solution but is a parameter, constant only for a particular temperature. Because of the tendency of gas molecules to seek the gaseous state when temperature rises, K_T varies inversely as a function of temperature.

The experimental determination of the solubility coefficient at several temperatures requires measurements of solution concentration (solubility) and partial pressure at each temperature. Technically, it is easier to measure the volume of gas that dissolves and calculate the number of moles of dissolved gas from the measured volume of dissolved gas, V, using the ideal gas law.

$$PV = n_L RT,$$

where:

P = the partial pressure of the gas in the gas phase,
V = the volume of gas dissolved in the liquid,
n_L = the number of moles of gas dissolved in the liquid,
R = the universal gas constant,
T = the absolute temperature,

and

$$n_L = \frac{PV}{RT}.$$

From Henry's law:

$$K_T = \frac{n_L}{PV_L}.$$

Substituting for n_L we get,

$$K_T = \frac{PV}{RTPV_L} = \left(\frac{1}{RT}\right)\left(\frac{V}{V_L}\right).$$

The quantity V/V_L is called the *Ostwald solubility coefficient* at temperature T and given the symbol λ_T (the Greek letter lambda). It is named after Wilhelm Ostwald (1853-1932), the German physical chemist. The Ostwald solubility coefficient is related to the solubility coefficient K_T by the above equation which may be restated as:

$$K_T = \frac{\lambda_T}{RT}$$

where:

K_T is the solubility coefficient at temperature T,
λ_T is the Ostwald solubility coefficient (at temperature T),
R is the universal gas constant,
T is the absolute temperature at which the experimental measurement of λ_T was performed.

The Ostwald solubility coefficient is a parameter, constant for any particular temperature, but varying inversely with some function of temperature. It is often used as an expression of solubility if the solution concentration is thought of as a volume per volume rather than a mass per unit volume. Defining the term solubility in this way means that Henry's law does not apply; this solubility is independent of pressure because although more gas dissolves with higher pressures, the volume shrinks according to Boyle's law. This solubility only varies inversely with some function of temperature.

In the experimental determination of λ_T the volume of dissolved gas is measured at the temperature, T, of the experiment. A further standardization of this volume can be made by reducing it to a standard temperature of 0°C (273 K) using Charles' law:

$$V(0°C) = \frac{V \cdot 273}{T},$$

where V is the volume of dissolved gas at an absolute temperature T, and $V(0°C)$ is the volume at 273 K, 0°C. The quantity $V(0°C)/V_L$ is called the *Bunsen solubility coefficient* at temperature T, and given the symbol α_T (the Greek letter alpha). It is named after Robert W. E. Bunsen (1811-1899), the German chemist. Its relation to the Ostwald solubility coefficient is

$$\alpha_T = \frac{\lambda_T \cdot 273}{T}$$

TABLE XV

OSTWALD SOLUBILITY COEFFICIENTS ($\lambda_{37°C}$)*

	Water	*Blood (Man)*	*Oil (Olive)*
Chloroform	3.8	10.3	265
Diethyl ether	15.61	15.2	50.2
N_2O	0.435	0.46	1.4
Trichloroethylene	1.55	9.15	—
Halothane	0.74	2.34	224
Methoxyflurane	4.5	13.0	825
Cyclopropane	0.204	0.415	11.2
Ethylene	0.081	0.140	1.28

* Larson, C. P. Jr., E. I. Eger and J. W. Severinghaus: The solubility of halothane in blood and tissue homogenates. *Anesthesiology, 23:*349-355, 1962.

Larson, C. P. Jr., E. I. Eger and J. W. Severinghaus: Ostwald solubility coefficients for anesthetic gases in various fluids and tissues. *Anesthesiology, 23:*686-689, 1962.

Eger, E. I. and R. Shargel: The solubility of methoxyflurane in human blood and tissue homogenates. *Anesthesiology, 24:*625-627, 1963.

and to the solubility coefficient K_T is

$$K_T = \frac{a_T}{R \cdot 273}.$$

Table XV lists some solubility coefficients of interest to anaesthetists.

As well as a practical expression of the solubility coefficient, the Ostwald solubility coefficient also has the useful property of being equal to the ratio of the concentrations (moles/volume) of the gas in dissolved and gaseous states. The relationship can be established as follows:

$$\lambda_T = \frac{V}{V_L}.$$

We know from the previous derivation that V is the volume occupied by n_L moles of dissolved gas, and that

$$V = \frac{n_L RT}{P}.$$

Therefore, substituting in the Ostwald solubility coefficient equation we get

$$\lambda_T = \frac{n_L RT}{V_L P},$$

and

$$\lambda_T = \frac{(n_L/V_L)}{(P/RT)}.$$

Now in the gaseous state, the ideal gas law states that

$$PV_G = n_G RT,$$

where:

P is the partial pressure,
V_G is the volume occupied by
n_G, the number of moles of gas not dissolved,

and

T is the absolute temperature.

Rearranging,

$$\frac{P}{RT} = \frac{n_G}{V_G}.$$

Substitute in the equation for the Ostwald solubility coefficient to get

$$\lambda_T = \frac{(n_L/V_L)}{(n_G/V_G)}.$$

That is to say, the Ostwald solubility coefficient may also be defined as the ratio of the concentrations (moles/litre) of the gas in dissolved and gaseous states.

The *partition coefficient* is somewhat similar to the above expression. It is the ratio of the concentrations of a gas dissolved in two different liquids, when equilibrium is established between both liquids and the gaseous state. The partition coefficient is particularly useful to express the distribution of an anaesthetic between lipid and blood at 37°C. Experimentally, this particular partition coefficient is approximated by shaking a mixture of the anaesthetic gas, water and vegetable oil until equilibrium is established and then, measuring the concentration of the gas in both liquids. The partition coefficient may also be calculated as the ratio of Ostwald solubility coefficients for each liquid. Like the other solubility coefficients, the partition coefficient is constant only for a particular temperature.

DIFFUSION

In the last section a solution was defined as a uniform intermingling of different kinds of molecules. The transfer of a substance from one location to another by a process of molecular intermingling is called *diffusion*. Several forces may operate to cause diffusion, for example, a pressure difference, an electrical field and a concentration difference.

Consider two fluid-filled compartments separated by a rigid wall through which the fluid can pass by a process of molecular intermingling. If the hydrostatic pressure on one side of the wall is higher than on the other then the fluid molecules will transfer to the low pressure side. If the molecules are charged, then an electric field applied across the wall will cause a transfer of molecules through the wall. If the fluid is a solution containing a substance whose concentration is different on each side of the wall, then the substance will transfer through the wall from the higher concentration to the lower.

The latter type of diffusion is responsible for the uniform intermingling of a solution and was studied by Adolph Eugen Fick (1829-1901), the German physiologist and medical physicist. He found it to obey the following law:

$$\frac{dM}{dt} \propto \frac{dC}{dx},$$

where:

M is the mass of a particular substance,
t is time,
C is the concentration of the substance,

and

x is distance along the diffusion pathway.

The term dM/dt is the diffusion flow of mass in a given time, and the term dC/dx is the slope of the graph of concentration along the diffusion path length x; dC/dx is often termed the concentration gradient.

Since anaesthetists are often concerned with the diffusion of gases in liquid solutions it is convenient to restate Fick's law in terms of partial pressure instead of concentration.

Fick's law may be converted to a form using the partial pressure gradient by the application of Henry's law which states that

$$C = K_T P.$$

Fick's Law for the diffusion of gases becomes

$$\frac{dM}{dt} \propto K_T \frac{dP}{dx},$$

where:

dM/dt = the diffusion flow,
dP/dx = the partial pressure gradient along the diffusion path,
K_T = the solubility coefficient of the gas in the medium in which the diffusion is taking place.

As well as applying to the diffusion of gas molecules in gaseous and liquid phases, Fick's law applies to the diffusion of gas molecules through membranes if the molecules flow through the membrane by a process of molecular intermingling in the structure of the membrane. Note that the flow of gases through porous membrane is termed *effusion* rather than diffusion. The process is somewhat different and not treated here.

In the case of a gas diffusing through a thin membrane such as that shown in Figure 47, the differential form of Fick's law solves to

$$\frac{M}{t} \propto \frac{K_T(P_1 - P_2)}{L},$$

where:

M/t = the average diffusion flow (mass per unit time),
$P_1 - P_2$ = the partial pressure difference across the membrane,

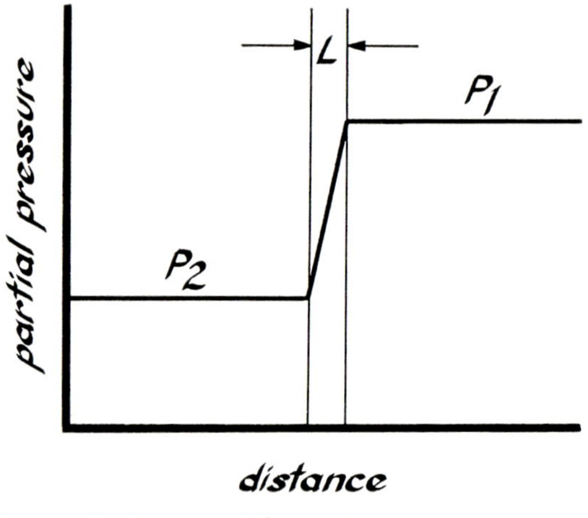

Figure 47. Gaseous diffusion through a membrane.

K_T = the solubility coefficient of the gas in the membrane,
L = the thickness of the membrane.

The diffusion flow is also proportional to the area of the membrane, A, so that in equation form Fick's law becomes,

$$\frac{M}{t} = \frac{D \cdot K_T \cdot A}{L} (P_1 - P_2),$$

where:

D = the constant of proportionality, called the *diffusivity* or the *diffusion constant* of the gas in the membrane material.

A membrane is said to be permeable to the particular gases whose molecules will diffuse through it, and the product of the constants $D \cdot K_T$ is called the *permeability*. Often the constants of the equation $D \cdot K_T \cdot A/L$ are lumped as one inclusive constant known as the *diffusing capacity*. The diffusing capacity can then be expressed in units of mass flow per unit pressure difference, such as moles per minutes per mm Hg. The equation becomes analogous to those for heat flow, fluid flow and electricity flow; with the diffusing capacity analogous to conductance, the reciprocal of resistance.

The membrane equation for the diffusion of gases shows that diffusion flow varies directly as the area of the membrane and inversely as the thickness. This dependence is readily comprehended; we would expect the diffusion flow to double for twice the area and to halve for twice the thickness. The diffusion flow is also dependent upon the solubility coefficient of the gas in the material of the membrane. This dependence occurs because the process of diffusion is also one of solution. For example, the high solubility of oxygen in silicone rubber as compared with that in plastics contributes to the success of silicone rubber as a membrane material for artificial lungs. Similarly, the high solubility of carbon dioxide in water as compared to that of oxygen in water contributes to the larger diffusion flow of carbon dioxide through an aqueous membrane (like the alveolar membrane) under identical partial pressure gradients.

The diffusion constant in the equation varies as a function of both the temperature and density of the gas. Since K.E. increases the motion of gas molecules, it is not unexpected to find that the diffusion flow increases as a function of temperature. Diffusion flow also depends upon a function of gas density.

Thomas Graham (1805-1869), the English chemist, studied the diffusion of gases, both through membranes and in solutions, and determined that the diffusion flow varied inversely as the square root of the density of the gas, providing the gradient was kept constant. *Graham's law* may be written as a ratio of the diffusion constants for gases 1 and 2. Given that

$$D \propto \frac{1}{\sqrt{\rho}},$$

then

$$\frac{D_1}{D_2} = \sqrt{\frac{\rho_2}{\rho_1}},$$

and if the two gases are at the same temperature and pressure, then

$$\frac{D_1}{D_2} = \sqrt{\frac{MW_2}{MW_1}}$$

where: MW = molecular weight.

It should also be noted that Graham's law applies not only to the diffusion of gases through membranes but also to the effusion of gases through porous membranes.

OSMOSIS

The selective diffusion of molecules through a semipermeable membrane is responsible for the effect called *osmosis*. Osmosis is the diffusion of solvent molecules through a membrane which is permeable to the solvent molecules but not to the solute molecules. The diffusion follows Fick's law, and solvent molecules transfer through the membrane from a region of high solvent concentration to a region of low solvent concentration. Consider a solution of glucose and water separated from pure water by a membrane permeable only to water as shown in Figure 48. The concentration gradient for water acts to cause the diffusion of water molecules through the membrane and into the glucose solution in a process of osmosis. The osmosis continues until equilibrium is attained. Either the concentrations on each side become equal (which cannot happen unless there is some glucose

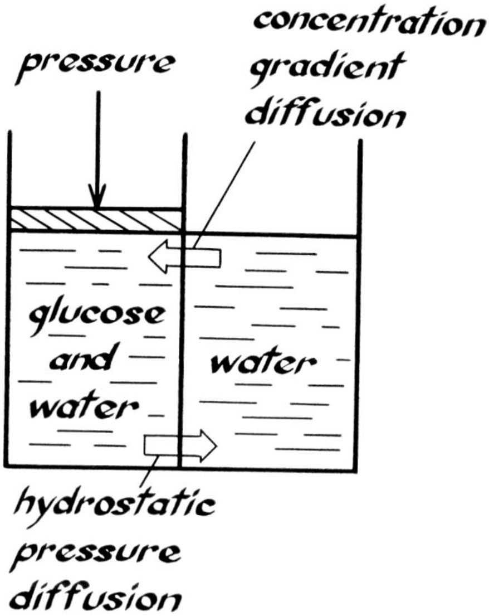

Figure 48. Definition of osmotic pressure.

on each side of the membrane), or the hydrostatic pressure of the glucose solution rises with respect to the water such that the pressure forces the water to diffuse back through the membrane as fast as it diffuses through due to osmosis. The hydrostatic pressure which is required to prevent a net transfer of water across the membrane is thought of as equal and opposite to the effect of the concentration gradient causing osmosis.

The *osmotic pressure* of a solution may, therefore, be defined as equal and opposite to the hydrostatic pressure which must be exerted on the solution to prevent the net diffusion of solvent, when the solution is separated from pure solvent by a membrane permeable only to solvent. Because the osmotic pressure depends upon the number of discrete particles in the solution rather than the size or type of molecule, solutes that ionize develop twice the osmotic pressure of unionized solutes at the same concentration. Solutions which develop the same osmotic pressure are termed isosmotic. Solutions containing more than one solute develop a total osmotic pressure equal to the sum of the osmotic pressures developed by each solute.

Living cells are surrounded by semipermeable membranes, and can therefore be destroyed by cell volume changes caused by osmosis. It is not enough, however, to control the osmotic pressure of solutions in contact with cell membranes, because the membranes are not only permeable to water (solvent) molecules but also to some solute molecules. The solute molecules that can diffuse through the membrane act as if they were solvent molecules and move accordingly, so that the pressure which may damage the cell membrane is due only to the unequal concentrations of the solute molecules that cannot pass through the membrane. The pressure developed by diffusion in these circumstances is called the *tone* of a solution. The tone of a solution may be defined as the hydrostatic pressure which must be exerted on the solution to prevent the net diffusion of the molecules to which the membrane is permeable, when the solution is separated from a solution made purely of molecules which can diffuse through the membrane. In other words, while the osmotic pressure of a solution is defined as being determined by the total concentration of solute molecules, the tone of a solution is determined by the concentration of those solute molecules that cannot pass through the membrane used in a particular situation. Solutions of the same tone are isotonic; lower tone, hypotonic; higher tone, hypertonic. As in the case of osmotic pressure, ionization doubles the osmotic effect. The clinical standard for tone is the contents of the red cell, which is isotonic with a sodium chloride solution of 0.9 grams per 100 ml H_2O.

PROBLEM 8

(a) The alveolar concentration of halothane in an anaesthetized patient was determined as 1% volume/volume. Estimate the brain and blood concentrations (in mol/l) of halothane. Assume that equilibrium has been reached between alveolar air, blood and brain tissue, and that brain tissue has the same solubility coefficient as oil.

(b) What concentration of glucose in water solution is isosmotic with a sodium chloride in water solution of 0.9 g/100 ml? The molecular weights of sodium chloride and glucose are 58 and 180 respectively. NaCl is 90 percent ionized.

(c) Solution A is separated from solution B by a semipermeable membrane which is permeable only to water and urea. In each of the following cases, compare the osmotic pressures (isosmotic or not?), and also the tone (hyper-, hypo-, or isotonic?) of the water solutions (B with respect to A).

	A	B
Case 1	glucose 1 mol/l	glycerin 1 mol/l
Case 2	glucose 1 mol/l	urea 1 mol/l
Case 3	urea 1 mol/l	glycerin 1 mol/l
Case 4	urea 1 mol/l and glycerin 1 mol/l	glucose 1 mol/l

(d) How much slower (%) than oxygen will nitrous oxide effuse through a rubber bag?

Chapter 9

FLUID MECHANICS

VISCOSITY

IN THE LAST CHAPTER, a fluid was defined as a substance that cannot sustain static shear forces. It can, however, sustain shear forces under dynamic conditions due to a property called *viscosity*. The flow of any fluid constitutes a continually increasing strain as the fluid layers slide past each other, and under these conditions a shearing force exists between the layers. These internal shearing forces are viscous forces, a sort of friction that results in the degradation of the mechanical energy of the flow into heat energy. Because the heat cannot be converted back into the form of mechanical energy, it is an energy loss. Viscosity is the property of a fluid which defines the extent of this energy loss.

According to the kinetic molecular theory, the action of viscous forces in a fluid that give rise to the property of viscosity may be regarded as a momentum exchange between adjacent fluid layers which have different velocities. The momentum exchange reduces the relative motion between neighbouring layers. To understand what is meant by momentum exchange, imagine two trains parallel to each other and moving in the same direction but at different speeds. A mass thrown from the slow train to the fast train will cause the fast train to slow down, while a mass thrown from the fast train to the slow train will cause the slow train to speed up. This momentum exchange between the two trains reduces the difference between their speeds.

In Chapter 8, we discussed the fact that the production of an elastic deformation or strain in a solid required that a shear stress be applied which is proportional to the strain. The linear portion of the stress versus strain graph is characterized by its slope, the ratio of shear stress to shear strain, which is called the *shear modulus*. Ideally, a fluid has a shear modulus of zero under static conditions because the fluid layers flow past each other to relieve the stress. During flow, however, the fluid layers do support a dynamic shear stress as the fluid layers slide by one another. The dynamic shear stress is given the symbol τ. Tau (τ) is proportional to the difference in velocity between the layers of the fluid. Because each layer could be subdivided into a number of thinner layers almost *ad infinitum,* the difference in velocity is expressed as a velocity difference per unit distance between the layers, and called the velocity gradient, or the rate of shearing strain. The velocity gradient is therefore the slope of a graph plotting the difference in velocity between layers versus their distance apart. Newton defined a dynamic shear modulus for fluids analogous to the shear modulus for solids. He called it *dynamic viscosity,* and it has the symbol μ (the Greek letter mu).

$$\mu = \frac{\text{shearing stress}}{\text{rate of shearing strain}}.$$

The concept of dynamic viscosity and its definition may be illustrated by considering the motion of a fluid between two plates as shown in Figure 49. The lower plate is stationary, and the upper plate is moved at a constant velocity U, which requires a force, F, to be exerted upon the plate. A very thin layer of fluid adheres to each of the plates because of molecular attraction.

It is assumed that the fluid forms a series of parallel layers (laminas) within which the velocity of the fluid is uniform, and that there are no secondary, irregular fluid motions or fluctua-

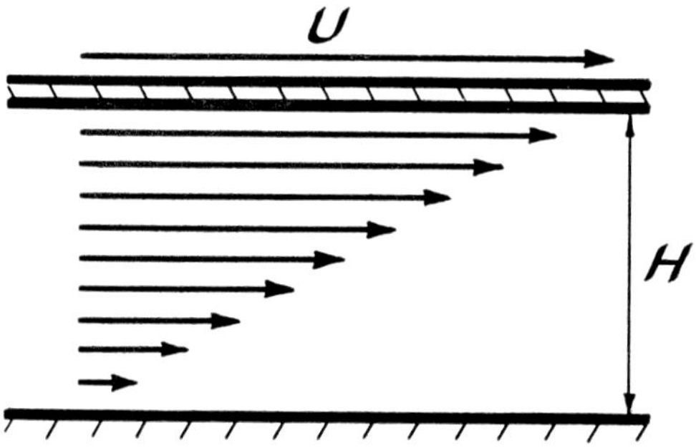

Figure 49. Definition of dynamic viscosity.

tions superimposed upon the fluid flow set up by the moving plate. Such flow is called *laminar flow.* The velocities of the fluid layers between the plates vary linearly with distance, from zero at the surface of the lower plate to U at the surface of the upper plate, a distance of H units away. A graph of this variation of fluid velocity versus distance is called a *velocity distribution.* For our example, it is a straight line, as Figure 49 demonstrates. The slope of the velocity distribution is called either the *velocity gradient* or the *rate of shearing strain,* and is equal to U/H in this example.

The dynamic viscosity of the fluid pictured in Figure 49 is therefore

$$\mu = \frac{\tau}{U/H}.$$

But τ, the shearing stress, is the force F applied over the area of the plate, A. So,

$$\mu = \frac{F/A}{U/H}.$$

In this example, the velocity distribution was linear so that the velocity gradient was constant throughout the fluid. Suppose that the velocity distribution was not linear. We would then find it necessary to express the velocity gradient as the slope of the velocity distribution at a particular point, that is as the derivative, du/dh. The stress developed between the two layers of fluid at that particular location in the fluid would then be

$$\tau = \mu \cdot \frac{du}{dh}.$$

The equation above shows that if the relation between shear stress, τ, and the velocity gradient, du/dh, is linear, then the slope μ is constant. Dynamic viscosity may, therefore, be thought of as a constant of proportionality, a property of a fluid. Fluids whose dynamic viscosity is a constant are called *Newtonian fluids.* Fluids, like blood, whose relationship between the shear stress and velocity gradient are nonlinear do not have a constant dynamic viscosity and are called non-Newtonian fluids.

The dimensions of dynamic viscosity in S.I. units can be

found from a dimensional analysis of the defining equation. Since shear stress is force per unit area (newtons per square metre), and the velocity gradient is velocity per unit distance (metres per second per metre), therefore

$$\mu = \frac{N/m^2}{m/s/m} = \frac{N \cdot s}{m^2} = Pa \cdot s.$$

The S.I. unit of dynamic viscosity is thus, the pascal-second, with the symbol Pa · s. In the older c.g.s. system of units, the unit of dynamic viscosity is the poise, named after Jean Léonard Marie Poiseuille (1799-1869), the French physiologist and physicist. Table XVI lists the dynamic viscosity of some fluids of interest to anaesthetists.

Dynamic viscosity is temperature dependent, as might be expected. It increases with temperature in gases and decreases with temperature in liquids. On a molecular scale, the interaction of gas molecules becomes greater as the temperature rises; the molecules have a higher K.E. so that the interaction or friction between laminas of gas is greater. Liquid molecules, in contrast, are primarily influenced by the fleeting, weak bonds which characterize a liquid. An increase in their K.E. serves to weaken the effect of these bonds, decreasing the interaction between laminas.

TABLE XVI

VISCOSITIES AND DENSITIES (μ, ρ)

Substance	μ *Pa · s*[1]	ρ *kg/m*^{3} *or g/l @ 760 mm Hg*[2]
Water	10^{-3} @ 20°C	10^3 @ 20°C
Mercury	1.685×10^{-3} @ 0°C	13.6×10^3 @ 0°C
Glycerin	12.11 @ 0°C	1.26×10^3 @ 0°C
Air	1.83×10^{-5} @ 20°C	1.2 @ 20°C
Oxygen (O_2)	2.036×10^{-5} @ 20°C	1.429 @ 0°C
Nitrogen (N_2)	1.781×10^{-5} @ 27.4°C	1.25 @ 0°C
Carbon dioxide	1.48×10^{-5} @ 20°C	1.976 @ 0°C
Nitrous oxide	1.49×10^{-5} @ 26.9°C	1.977 @ 0°C
Helium	1.94×10^{-5} @ 20°C	0.164 @ 0°C

[1] Robert C. Weast (Ed.): *Handbook of Chemistry and Physics*, 54th Edition. Chemical Rubber Company Press, Cleveland, Ohio, U.S.A., 1973-1974.

[2] Paul G. Stecker (Ed.): *The Merck Index*. Merck and Company Ltd., Rahway, New Jersey, U.S.A.

Kinematic viscosity is defined as the ratio of dynamic viscosity to density:

$$\nu = \frac{\mu}{\rho},$$

where:

ν = kinematic viscosity (the Greek letter nu),
μ = dynamic viscosity,
ρ = density.

The usefulness of this definition will become evident later in this chapter. A dimensional analysis,

$$\nu = \frac{\text{Pa} \cdot \text{s}}{\text{kg/m}^3} = \frac{\text{N} \cdot \text{s/m}^2}{\text{kg/m}^3} = \frac{\text{kg} \cdot \text{m} \cdot \text{s/m}^2 \cdot \text{s}^2}{\text{kg/m}^3},$$

$$\nu = \text{m}^2/\text{s},$$

demonstrates that the S.I. unit of kinematic viscosity is the square metre per second. In the c.g.s. system, the unit of kinematic viscosity, cm^2/s, has been named the stoke, after Sir George Gabriel Stokes (1819-1903), the English mathematician and physicist.

REYNOLDS NUMBER

There are two main types of fluid flow; laminar and turbulent. In laminar flow, the fluid moves in thin layers or laminas as in the previous example, while in *turbulent flow* secondary irregular motions and velocity fluctuations are superimposed upon the average flow. Smoke rising in a calm atmosphere often demonstrates these two types of flow. Immediately above the source of the smoke, the smoke rises in smooth filaments which may wave about but do not lose their identity; this flow is laminar and dominated by viscous friction forces. At some distance above the source, the laminar flow suddenly breaks into a confused eddying motion; this flow is turbulent and dominated by momentum forces. In turbulent flow the velocity of the smoke upwards has become so great that, instead of flowing smoothly together in an orderly flow held together by viscous friction forces, the smoke follows a course determined by the momentum of the individual particles.

From this example, it can be seen that the ratio of the forces due to viscous friction and the forces due to momentum characterize the flow of a fluid because it determines which type of flow is more likely to occur in any given situation.

Anaesthetists are concerned with flow in tubes and pipes, in other words, in completely enclosed volumes. Consider the flow of a fluid in a tube of circular cross section. At the interior surface of the pipe, a very thin layer of fluid adheres to the pipe wall and has zero velocity. Along the central axis of the tube the velocity is a maximum. In laminar flow the velocity distribution is parabolic in profile, varying from zero velocity at the pipe walls to a maximum at the axis in a series of laminas concentric with the axis of the tube. Figure 50 shows the velocity distribution as a two dimensional graph called a *velocity profile.* The velocity distribution for the turbulent flow can only be approximated because of the random fluctuation in local flows, but it has been measured and is the shape of a flattened parabola, as shown in Figure 50.

It is important for the anaesthetist to be able to predict the type of flow in any given situation, not only because of changes in the boundary layer, but also because pressure losses increase markedly for turbulent flow. For fluids flowing in tubes, an index of behaviour called the *Reynolds number* (symbol N_R) is used to predict the type of flow that will result for any given flow and tubing. The index of behaviour is named after its inventor, Osborne Reynolds (1842-1912), the English physicist and engineer, and is the ratio of the force of momentum within the fluid to the force of viscous friction.

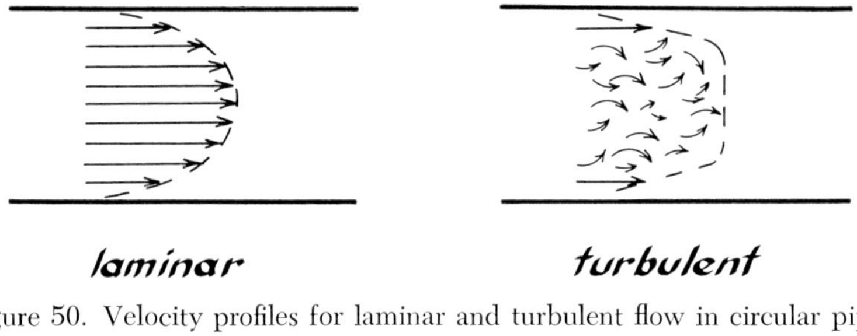

Figure 50. Velocity profiles for laminar and turbulent flow in circular pipes.

The average force due to momentum within the fluid is the average rate of change of momentum with time, that is

$$\text{momentum force} = \frac{M\bar{v}}{t},$$

where:

> M is the mass of a characteristic volume of fluid,
> $\bar{v}$ is the average fluid velocity,
> t is a characteristic time interval.

The time, t, can be considered as the time taken for the fluid to move along a characteristic length of tubing, say L. Therefore,

$$t = \frac{L}{\bar{v}}.$$

The mass of a characteristic volume of fluid, V, is the product of that volume and the density of the fluid, that is

$$M = V\rho \propto D^2L\rho,$$

where: D is the diameter of the tubing.

We conclude that the momentum force is proportional to

$$\frac{D^2L\rho\bar{v}}{L/\bar{v}} = \rho D^2\bar{v}^2$$

The viscous friction force within the fluid is proportional to the viscous shear stress, τ, applied over a characteristic area of the fluid, such as a segment of the tubing wall which is proportional to D^2. So

$$\text{viscous force} \propto \tau D^2.$$

Now, since

$$\tau = \mu \frac{du}{dh},$$

and the velocity gradient, du/dh, is proportional to $\bar{v}/D$, then,

$$\tau \propto \frac{\mu\bar{v}}{D},$$

and the viscous force is proportional to

$$\frac{\mu\bar{v}}{D} \cdot D^2 = \mu\bar{v}D.$$

Reynolds number, the ratio of the momentum force to the viscous force is

$$N_R = \frac{\rho D^2 \bar{v}^2}{\mu \bar{v} D} = \frac{D \bar{v} \rho}{\mu} = \frac{D \bar{v}}{\nu},$$

where:

N_R = the Reynolds number,
D = the diameter of the tube,
$\bar{v}$ = the average velocity of the fluid,
ρ = the density of the fluid,
μ = the dynamic viscosity of the fluid,
ν = the kinematic viscosity of the fluid.

The following dimensional analysis demonstrates that the Reynolds number is an index of behaviour and has no units:

$$N_R = \frac{D\bar{v}}{\nu} = \frac{\text{m} \cdot \text{m/s}}{\text{m}^2/\text{s}} = \frac{\text{m}^2/\text{s}}{\text{m}^2/\text{s}}.$$

However, the calculation of Reynolds number must still, of course, be carried out using a consistent system of units.

The nature of any particular flow of a fluid may be judged to some extent from the corresponding Reynolds number; a small number indicates that viscous forces predominate, and flow is laminar. Whereas a large number shows that momentum forces have more effect, and flow is turbulent. For example, for a given flow, mercury with a high density and correspondingly high N_R would tend to turbulence more than glycerin with a high viscosity and low N_R.

Experiments have shown that the stable form of motion for fluid flowing in a tube is normally laminar for $N_R < 2000$. Below $N_R = 2000$, an initially turbulent flow cannot be maintained indefinitely and becomes laminar. Above $N_R = 4000$ flow is turbulent. This experimental determination will be used later in this chapter to develop a test for laminar flow.

THE EQUATION OF CONTINUITY

The equation of continuity is an application of the general law of conservation of matter. It simply states that if a tube is completely full of a steadily flowing fluid, then the mass flow

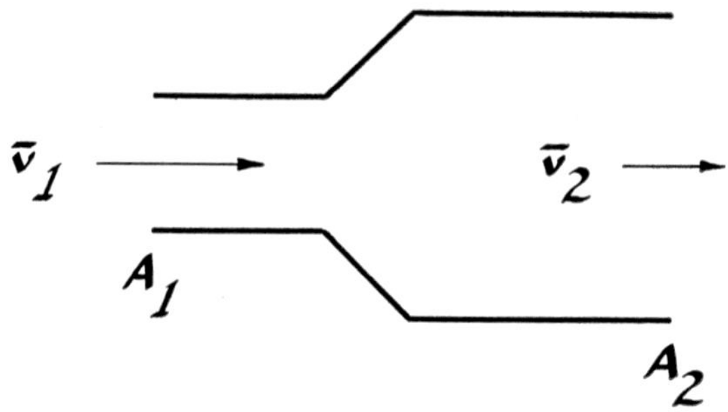

Figure 51. Illustration of the equation of continuity.

past one point in the tube must equal the mass flow past another point in the tube.

Figure 51 shows a fluid flowing through a tube whose cross-sectional area changes from A_1 to A_2. At section 1, the average velocity $\bar{v}_1$ is L_1/t; length L_1 is traversed in time t. The volume of fluid V_1, which passes in time t is therefore

$$F = \frac{V_1}{t} = \frac{L_1 A_1}{t} = A_1 \bar{v}_1.$$

Note that F is used to denote fluid flow here. It is similar to the symbols $\dot{V}$ and $\dot{Q}$ which anaesthetists use to represent the specific flows of gas and blood respectively. The correct definition of F is dV/dt, but in this case the flow is steady and the average flow V/t is equal to dV/dt.

The mass of fluid passing section 1 per unit time is

$$\frac{V_1}{t} \cdot \rho_1 = A_1 \bar{v}_1 \rho_1,$$

where: ρ_1 is the density of the fluid at section 1.
Similarly, the mass of fluid passing section 2 per unit time is $A_2 \bar{v}_2 \rho_2$.

The equation of continuity states that these two mass flows must be equal so

$$A_1 \bar{v}_1 \rho_1 = A_2 \bar{v}_2 \rho_2.$$

If the density of the fluid is unchanged between sections 1 and 2, then $\rho_1 = \rho_2$ and

$$A_1 \bar{v}_1 = A_2 \bar{v}_2 = F.$$

The equation simply states a reciprocal dependence between cross-sectional area and flow velocity. The circulation of blood provides an example of this dependence; for any given cardiac output the velocity of blood flow in the aorta is much greater than that in the capillaries because the total cross-sectional area of all capillaries is many times larger than that of the aorta.

THE GENERAL ENERGY EQUATION

The general energy equation considers the energy relationships of a steadily flowing fluid with its surroundings. The equation itself looks very complicated but is merely a large number of simple relationships. Recalling the relationship between work and energy as set out in Chapter 4, examine the energy relationships shown in Figure 52 as a fluid enters a tube at section 1, and leaves it at section 2.

At each section the fluid will possess energy: P.E. with respect to the earth's gravitational field, K.E., the energy of motion, and internal energy (molecular P.E. and K.E.).

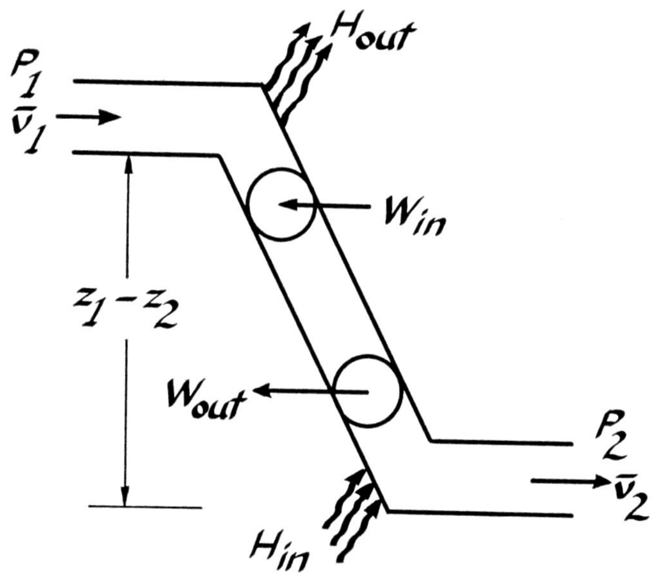

Figure 52. Energy relationships of a steadily flowing fluid with its surroundings.

Between sections 1 and 2 energy may be added or subtracted from the fluid in several ways. Mechanical work may be done on the fluid (a ventilator for example), and mechanical work may be done by the fluid (turning a Wright respirometer for example); the addition and subtraction of energy respectively. Similarly energy may be added or subtracted in the form of heat.

The law of conservation of energy states that energy is neither created nor destroyed in such a situation. The difference in the energy possessed by the fluid at sections 1 and 2 must equal the difference in the energy added and the energy subtracted between sections 1 and 2.

We can express the law quantitatively by examining the energy relationships of a unit mass of fluid, M.

The work done on the fluid pushing it into section 1 is the force per unit mass times the distance moved, that is

$$\frac{P_1 A_1}{M} \cdot \frac{V_1}{A_1} = \frac{P_1 V_1}{M}$$

where: P_1 = the fluid pressure at section 1,
A_1 = the cross-sectional area at section 1,
V_1 = the volume of the unit mass of fluid at section 1,
M = the unit mass of fluid.

but since M/V_1 is the density of the fluid at section 1, the work done is

$$\frac{P_1}{\rho_1}.$$

Similarly, the work done by the fluid pushing a unit mass out of section 2 is

$$\frac{P_2}{\rho_2}.$$

Let the mechanical work done on the fluid per unit mass, and the mechanical work done by the fluid per unit mass be

$$W_{IN} \text{ and } W_{OUT}$$

respectively.

Let the heat added and extracted per unit mass between sections 1 and 2 be

$$H_{IN} \text{ and } H_{OUT}$$

respectively.

Let the difference in the P.E. between sections 1 and 2 be

$$Z_1 - Z_2$$

per unit mass.

The K.E. possessed by a unit mass of the fluid at section 1 is equal to the work done on the fluid mass in giving it its average velocity, $\bar{v}_1$, at section 1, that is, work = force · distance. In this case the force required to give the fluid a final velocity of $\bar{v}_1$ is,

$$Ma = M\bar{v}_1/t.$$

The distance travelled in accelerating the fluid from zero velocity to $\bar{v}_1$ in time t is $t \cdot \bar{v}_1/2$ and so the K.E. possessed by the fluid at section 1, per unit mass, is

$$\frac{M\bar{v}_1}{t} \cdot \frac{t\bar{v}_1}{2} \cdot \frac{1}{M} = \frac{\bar{v}_1^2}{2}$$

and that at section 2 is

$$\frac{\bar{v}_2^2}{2}.$$

The internal energies per unit mass at sections 1 and 2 are

$$I_1 \text{ and } I_2$$

respectively.

Now that the necessary symbols have been defined we can add up the energies at 1 and 2, the energy added between 1 and 2, and the energy extracted. The energy per unit mass at section 1 is:

$$\frac{v_1^2}{2} + Z_1 + I_1,$$

and at section 2 is

$$\frac{\bar{v}_2^2}{2} + Z_2 + I_2.$$

The energy added to the fluid between sections 1 and 2 is

$$\frac{P_1}{\rho_1} + W_{IN} + H_{IN},$$

and the energy subtracted is

$$\frac{P_2}{\rho_2} + W_{OUT} + H_{OUT}.$$

The general energy equation is therefore:
(energy at 2) – (energy at 1) = (energy added) – (energy subtracted), and in symbols,

$$\left(\frac{\bar{v}_2^2}{2} + Z_2 + I_2\right) - \left(\frac{\bar{v}_1^2}{2} + Z_1 + I_1\right)$$

$$= \left(\frac{P_1}{\rho_1} + W_{IN} + H_{IN}\right) - \left(\frac{P_2}{\rho_2} + W_{OUT} + H_{OUT}\right).$$

Now this equation applies to virtually any situation. However, we can simplify it by assuming a situation encountered in anaesthetic practice. Make the following assumptions:

1. no mechanical energy transfer, that is

$$W_{IN} - W_{OUT} = 0.$$

2. no external heating, that is

$$H_{IN} = 0.$$

3. no change in fluid density, that is $\rho_1 = \rho_2 = \rho$.
4. since there is no change in density, there is therefore, no change in the internal energy; the fluid temperature remains constant and no change of state occurs, that is

$$I_1 - I_2 = 0.$$

5. no change in height between sections 1 and 2, that is

$$Z_1 - Z_2 = 0.$$

With these assumptions applied, we may reduce the general energy equation to a more manageable size, and it becomes

$$\frac{\bar{v}_2^2 - \bar{v}_1^2}{2} = \frac{P_1 - P_2}{\rho} - H_{OUT}.$$

Since the temperature of the fluid remains constant, and no heat is added, then H_{OUT} becomes the heat lost due to the internal friction of the flowing fluid.

$$H_{OUT} = \left(\frac{P_1 - P_2}{\rho}\right) - \left(\frac{\bar{v}_2^2 - \bar{v}_1^2}{2}\right).$$

If the friction loss per unit mass, H_{OUT}, is negligible, then the general energy equation becomes

$$\frac{P_1}{\rho} + \frac{\bar{v}_1^2}{2} - \frac{P_2}{\rho} - \frac{\bar{v}_2^2}{2} = 0,$$

or

$$\frac{P_1}{\rho} + \frac{\bar{v}_1^2}{2} = \frac{P_2}{\rho} + \frac{\bar{v}_2^2}{2} = \text{constant.}$$

Both forms of the general energy equation, the frictionless and that including friction, will prove useful in the next chapter.

PROBLEM 9

Water flows steadily at a flow of 60 1/min. in a horizontal tube of circular cross-section whose inside diameter changes from 2 cm to 4 cm (see Figure 51). The pressure in the 2 cm diameter section is measured as 5 mm Hg gauge. What is the pressure in the 4 cm diameter section, assuming no friction loss, and a negligible change in water density?

Chapter 10

APPLICATIONS OF FLUID MECHANICS

VENTURI INJECTORS

THE VENTURI INJECTOR is a gas powered device for producing either suction or diluted gas mixtures. It is based upon the principles of flow behaviour as described by the general energy equation. Figure 53 shows a simple, streamlined venturi tube consisting of a converging portion, a throat and a diverging portion.

Assuming a frictionless fluid whose density is constant, the relation between the pressure and average velocity at the inlet, P_i and $\bar{v}_i$, to the pressure and average velocity at the throat, P_t and $\bar{v}_t$, will be given by the frictionless form of the general energy equation.

$$\frac{P_i}{\rho} + \frac{\bar{v}_i^2}{2} = \frac{P_t}{\rho} + \frac{\bar{v}_t^2}{2}.$$

From the continuity equation,

$$F = A_i\bar{v}_i = A_t\bar{v}_t,$$

where:

A_i = the cross-sectional area of the inlet,
A_t = the cross-sectional area of the throat.

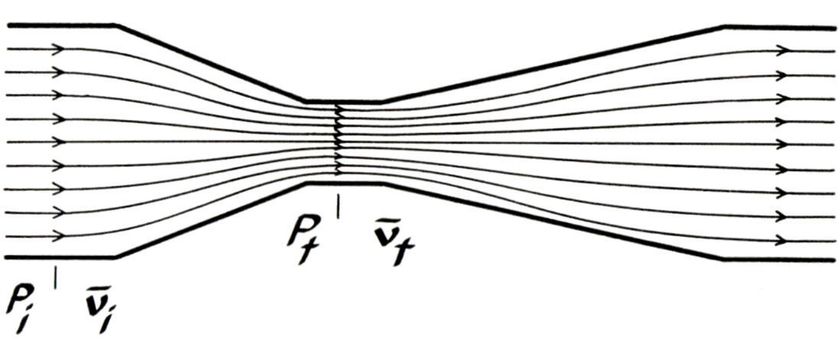

Figure 53. Venturi tube.

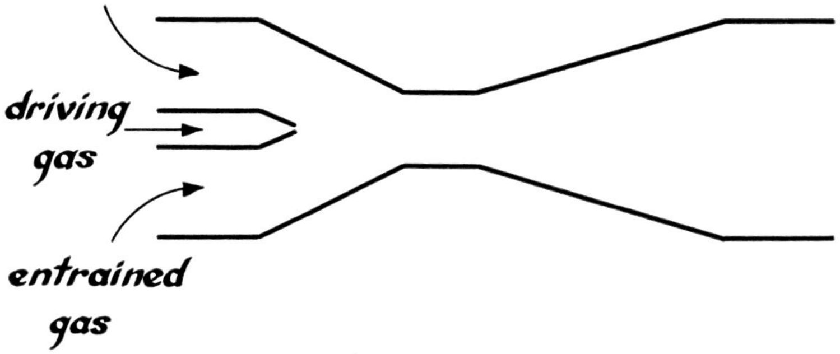

Figure 54. Venturi injector.

Therefore:

$$\bar{v}_t = \left(\frac{A_i}{A_t}\right) \bar{v}_i.$$

Substitute for $\bar{v}_t$ in the general energy equation to get,

$$\frac{P_i}{\rho} + \frac{\bar{v}_i^2}{2} = \frac{P_t}{\rho} + \left(\frac{A_i}{A_t}\right)^2 \cdot \frac{\bar{v}_i^2}{2}.$$

Solving for $P_i - P_t$:

$$\frac{P_i}{\rho} - \frac{P_t}{\rho} = \left(\frac{A_i}{A_t}\right)^2 \cdot \frac{\bar{v}_i^2}{2} - \frac{\bar{v}_i^2}{2},$$

and

$$P_i - P_t = \frac{\rho \bar{v}_i^2}{2}\left[\left(\frac{A_i}{A_t}\right)^2 - 1\right].$$

The equation above states that if $A_i > A_t$, then $P_t < P_i$. In other words, there has been an exchange of energy between pressure at the inlet and velocity at the throat. The energy at each position is the same.

Although this development is for the ideal case, a frictionless fluid of unchanging density, and is far from the real case of a gas with friction losses and a density dependent upon pressure, nevertheless it demonstrates the principle of operation of the venturi injector. Figure 54 shows a practical injector.

Figure 54 shows that the injector is a venturi tube with a nozzle concentric with the suction inlet; both occupying the inlet position of a venturi tube. In this configuration the entrainment of gas from the suction inlet is produced not only by the low pressure developed in the throat, but also by the propulsive effect of the gas jetting from the nozzle.

In a well designed injector the flow into the suction inlet is greater than the driving flow. The injector performance is rated according to its entrainment ratio, the ratio of driving gas flow to entrained gas flow. Because the entrainment ratio is less than one and relatively independent of flow the injector may be used to supply oxygen enriched air by driving the injector with oxygen and entraining air. If a valve is fitted to the suction inlet, the entrainment ratio may be set at a particular value so as to obtain the desired composition of the mixture. Since the composition is relatively unaffected by the injector flow, the injector may be used to supply specific gas mixtures intermittently, and is used for this purpose in some ventilators.

LAMINAR FLOW RESISTANCE

The term flow resistance is used to describe the property of a tube or pipe which causes an energy loss due to viscous friction in a flowing fluid. The energy loss is manifested as a pressure loss along the length of flow. From the general energy equation including viscous friction, the energy loss per unit mass of fluid is

$$H_{OUT} = \frac{P_1 - P_2}{\rho} - \frac{\bar{v}_2^2 - \bar{v}_1^2}{2}.$$

For the particular case of tubing with a constant cross-sectional area, the continuity equation states that:

$$\bar{v}_1 = \bar{v}_2,$$

and so the general energy equation simplifies to

$$H_{OUT} = \frac{P_1 - P_2}{\rho}.$$

The equation states that the energy lost in a flowing fluid due to viscous friction manifests itself as a loss of pressure. This situation is analogous to the flow of electricity through a resistance where the resistance causes a fall in voltage. Thus, we think of a length of tubing as offering a resistance to flow, and as being a flow resistance.

We can intuitively guess that the viscous frictional dissipation of heat energy will increase directly with tubing length and inversely with tubing diameter. It is also perhaps understandable that the greater the velocity of flow and hence the K.E., the greater will be the frictional dissipation. In symbols,

$$\text{friction} \propto \frac{L}{D} \cdot \frac{\bar{v}^2}{2},$$

and so

$$\frac{P_1 - P_2}{\rho} = f \cdot \frac{L}{D} \cdot \frac{\bar{v}^2}{2},$$

where: f = the constant of proportionality called the friction coefficient.

From experimental work it has been found that for fully developed laminar flow in circular tubes,

$$f = \frac{64}{N_R}.$$

The friction loss equation becomes

$$\frac{P_1 - P_2}{\rho} = \frac{64}{N_R} \cdot \frac{L}{D} \cdot \frac{\bar{v}^2}{2},$$

and since

$$N_R = \frac{D\rho\bar{v}}{\mu},$$

substitution yields

$$\frac{P_1 - P_2}{\rho} = \frac{64\mu L\bar{v}^2}{D\rho\bar{v}D2},$$

and

$$P_1 - P_2 = \frac{32\mu L\bar{v}}{D^2}.$$

The equation above is called the *Hagen-Poiseuille law* after Gotthilf Heinrich Hagen (1797-1884), the German hydraulic engineer and Jean Léonard Marie Poiseuille (1799-1869), the French physiologist. The law applies only if:

1. no mechanical energy is transferred to or from the fluid,
2. the internal energy of the fluid is unchanged,

3. the density of the fluid remains constant,
4. the tubing diameter is fixed,
5. the tubing is level,
6. the flow is laminar.

These limitations are apparent through the development of the equation, thereby justifying its presentation. We can see that the limitations of the Hagen-Poiseuille law mean that it may apply to liquid flow but is at best an approximation to gas flow.

The Hagen-Poiseuille law may be expressed in terms of flow, F, instead of velocity by applying the equation of continuity,

$$F = A\bar{v},$$

where:

$$A = \frac{\pi D^2}{4} \text{ for circular tubes.}$$

Then,

$$P_1 - P_2 = \frac{128\ \mu LF}{\pi D^4}.$$

Finally, we may derive a formula for laminar flow resistance in circular tubes as

$$R = \frac{P_1 - P_2}{F} = \frac{128\ \mu L}{\pi D^4}.$$

Throughout the preceding development it is assumed that a consistent set of units such as the S.I. is used. If other units are used, then the appropriate correction factors must be applied. For example, the resistance equation could be stated as

$$R = \frac{16\ \mu L}{\pi D^4},$$

where:

R = resistance in mm Hg/litres/min.,
μ = fluid viscosity in Pascal-seconds,
L = tubing length in centimetres,
D = tubing diameter in centimetres.

From this section of development we conclude that in laminar flow, where viscous friction predominates, the resistance is a constant depending upon the geometry of the tubing and the viscosity of the fluid. The equations show that the diameter of the tubing is a crucial factor in determining the flow resistance since $R \propto 1/D^4$. This dependence means that to increase flow in a transfusion set, for example, it is more effective to use a larger bore needle than to raise the bottle to increase the pressure.

Because the above equations apply only to laminar flow, it is necessary to test each situation by calculating the Reynolds number. If the Reynolds number is below 2000, then the flow is laminar. Other tests may be developed from this condition such as the determination of a critical flow velocity, above which flow is turbulent.

Since

$$N_R = \frac{D \cdot \bar{v}_c \cdot \rho}{\mu} = 2000$$

at the critical point. Then the critical velocity, $\bar{v}_c$, is

$$\bar{v}_c = \frac{2000\ \mu}{D\rho},$$

and from the equation of continuity,

$$F_c = A\bar{v}_c,$$

where

$$A = \frac{\pi D^2}{4}.$$

We can determine a critical flow, F_c,

$$F_c = \frac{2000\ \mu\pi D^2}{4D\rho} = \frac{500\ \mu\pi D}{\rho}.$$

By using the appropriate units and correction factors, the following critical flows, below which flow is laminar, may be determined.

For air at 20°C and 760 mm Hg,

$$F_c = 14\ D,$$

where:

F_c = the critical flow in l/min.,
D = the diameter of the tube in cm.

For water at 20°C and 760 mm Hg,

$$F_c = 94\ D,$$

where:

F_c = the critical flow in ml/min.,
D = the diameter of the tube in mm.

TURBULENT FLOW RESISTANCE

At Reynolds numbers below 2000 flow is wholly laminar, and at Reynolds numbers greater than 4000 flow is turbulent. In between, there is a transition range where flow is partly laminar and partly turbulent. These limits apply to fluids flowing in long, constant diameter tubes, but in anaesthetic circuits there may be junctions, abrupt changes in diameter at connections and valves, as well as abrupt changes in flow direction. All of these circumstances induce turbulence, and so turbulent flow may exist in a circuit whose Reynolds number appears to indicate laminar flow. The reason for concern about turbulent flow is that turbulent flow resistance is much larger than laminar flow resistance. Consequently, apparatus designed for low flow resistance must avoid the incidence of turbulent flow.

For laminar flow resistance we derived a resistance equation for the quantitative determination of resistance. Fluid mechanics engineers apply a similar approach to turbulent flow, but the situation is complicated by the fact that the friction coefficient in turbulent flow is not simply a linear function of Reynolds number but a nonlinear function of both Reynolds number, and the surface roughness of the tubing walls. Although empirical expressions for friction coefficients do exist for standard industrial tubes and piping, they are of little use to the anaesthetist. For this reason the approach used to express turbulent flow resistance in anaesthesia is an empirical one, measuring and plotting the pressure loss versus flow relationship for particular situations.

Despite the use of empirical methods we can still gain understanding by examining the turbulent flow situation using the general energy equation. Figure 55 shows a length of tubing containing an orifice which induces turbulence into an otherwise laminar flow. Because of the high velocities and shearing rates in the swirling turbulence, the energy loss due to viscous friction is high, much higher than for laminar flow.

Consider the effect of the orifice if the fluid was frictionless. The orifice would act like a sort of elementary venturi tube, and

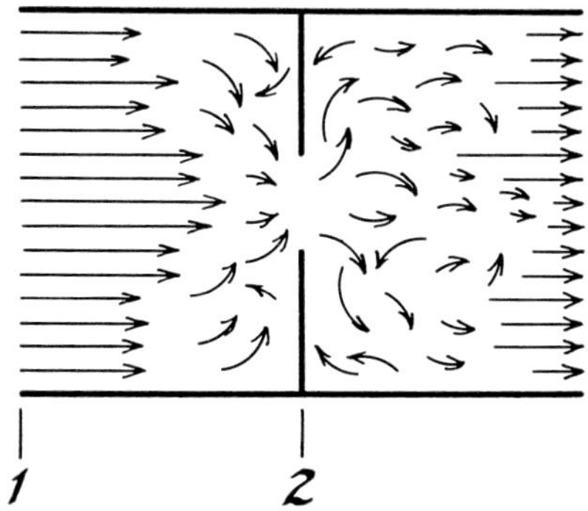

Figure 55. Flow through an orifice.

the pressure in the turbulence just after the orifice would be lowered relative to the pressure upstream from the orifice; the decreased pressure resulting from the increased velocities of the turbulence. If we can assume that the pressure loss in this frictionless case is proportional to the pressure loss in the real viscous friction case, then the general energy equation can be used to find an expression for turbulent flow resistance. From the frictionless form of the general energy equation, we can state that,

$$\frac{P_1}{\rho} + \frac{\bar{v}_1^2}{2} = \frac{P_2}{\rho} + \frac{\bar{v}_2^2}{2},$$

where the subscripts refer to sections 1 and 2, before and at the orifice respectively.

The continuity equation states that

$$F = A_1\bar{v}_1 = A_2\bar{v}_2,$$

where A_1 and A_2 are the cross-sectional areas of the tube and orifice respectively. Therefore

$$\bar{v}_1 = \left(\frac{A_2}{A_1}\right)\bar{v}_2,$$

and

$$\bar{v}_1^2 = \left(\frac{A_2}{A_1}\right)^2\bar{v}_2^2.$$

Substituting in the general energy equation for $\bar{v}_1^2$ yields

$$\frac{P_1}{\rho} + \left(\frac{A_2}{A_1}\right)^2 \cdot \frac{\bar{v}_2^2}{2} = \frac{P_2}{\rho} + \frac{\bar{v}_2^2}{2},$$

and

$$\frac{P_1 - P_2}{\rho} = \frac{\bar{v}_2^2}{2} - \left(\frac{A_2}{A_1}\right)^2 \cdot \frac{\bar{v}_2^2}{2},$$

and

$$P_1 - P_2 = \frac{\rho\bar{v}_2^2}{2}\left[1 - \left(\frac{A_2}{A_1}\right)^2\right].$$

From the continuity equation:

$$F = A_2\bar{v}_2,$$

and

$$\bar{v}_2 = \frac{F}{A_2}.$$

Substituting in the pressure loss equation:

$$P_1 - P_2 = \frac{\rho F^2}{2A_2^2}\left[1 - \left(\frac{A_2}{A_1}\right)^2\right],$$

and

$$R \propto \frac{P_1 - P_2}{F} = \frac{\rho F}{2A_2^2}\left[1 - \left(\frac{A_2}{A_1}\right)^2\right].$$

From the above equation we conclude that turbulent flow resistance is not only dependent upon the geometry of the flow situation but also dependent upon the flow itself. Turbulent resistance is not a constant but varies with flow. Also contrasting with the laminar flow resistance is the dependence of turbulent flow resistance upon fluid density rather than viscosity. The following table contrasts the behaviour characterizing laminar and turbulent flow resistances:

laminar	turbulent
R = constant	$R \propto F$
$P_1 - P_2 \propto F$	$P_1 - P_2 \propto F^2$
$R \propto \mu$	$R \propto \rho$

The development above demonstrates why the idea of resistance is discarded for turbulent flow and why measurements and graphs of pressure loss versus flow are used instead. Since the relationship between pressure loss and flow is nonlinear, curves and their equations are used. For example, a flow situation can be characterized for both laminar and turbulent flow by the equation:

$$P_1 - P_2 = C_1F + C_2F^2.$$

C_1 and C_2 are constants for the particular fluid and geometry. The first expression, C_1F, represents the pressure loss due to viscous friction in laminar flow, and the second expression, C_2F^2, represents the pressure lost in the viscous friction of turbulence. C_1 is a laminar flow resistance, but C_2 is not a flow resistance in the correct sense.

Another equation which may be used is

$$P_1 - P_2 = KF^n$$

where K and n are the constants for the particular situation. This equation does not apply throughout the whole flow range because $n = 1$ in laminar flow, $n = 2$ in turbulent flow, and is somewhere between 1 and 2 in transition cases. Nevertheless, the equation is useful for a limited range of flows.

The pressure loss versus flow relationship can be presented graphically as well as algebraically. Logarithmic scales are often used because a wide range of values can be covered. It is also

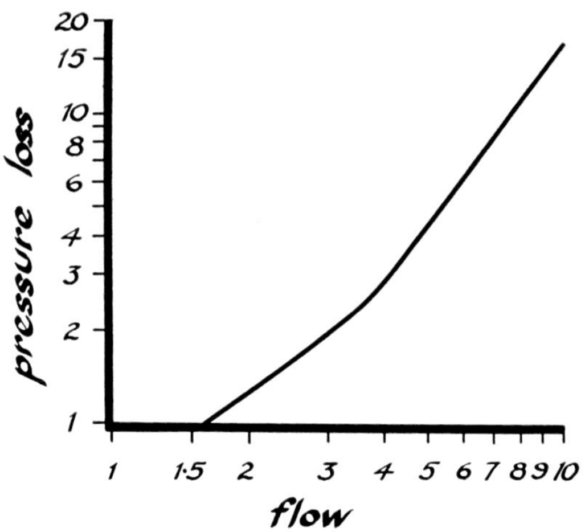

Figure 56. Typical logarithmic plot of pressure loss versus fluid flow for a section of a flow pathway.

useful to have a logarithmic plot because the graph slope is 1 for laminar flow and 2 for turbulent flow, and so these conditions are readily identified. Figure 56 shows a theoretical example.

GAS FLOWMETERS

There are two main types of flowmeter in use in anaesthesia; those using a fixed resistance, measuring the pressure loss; and those using a fixed pressure loss, measuring the position of a variable resistance which provides the pressure loss.

The first type of flowmeter uses a laminar flow resistance and is called the *pneumotachograph.* It is perhaps the most versatile gas meter since it is capable of recording rapidly changing flows. The pneumotachograph is based upon the measurement of the pressure difference across a laminar flow resistance. In accordance with the Hagen-Poiseuille law, the pressure drop is directly proportional to flow. Figure 57 shows a sketch of a pneumotachograph whose resistance is a strip of corrugated metal rolled into a tube.

The pressure difference is measured with a sensitive transducer which converts the pressure drop into electrical voltage. Since only a few mm H_2O pressure are needed to register a signal, the resistance offered by the flowmeter is negligible.

Because the pressure difference depends upon the viscosity of the gas, the pneumotachograph must be calibrated for each gas

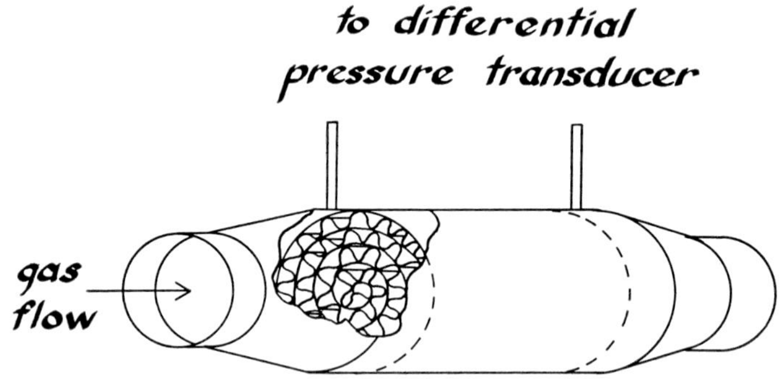

Figure 57. Pneumotachograph.

or gas mixture to be measured. For accurate measurements the pneumotachograph may be heated to a constant temperature because viscosity is temperature dependent. The heating has a further advantage in that it avoids condensation from saturated expired gas which could change the resistance.

The anaesthetist often wants to know the accumulated volume of gas rather than gas flow, and so these flowmeter signals are often connected to an electronic integrator. From the flowmeter we get

$$F = \frac{dV}{dt},$$

and the integrator provides

$$\int \frac{dV}{dt} = V.$$

If an electronic integrator is not available, the area beneath the flow (F) versus time graph may be measured to get volume (V). An instrument called a planimeter is used to measure areas enclosed by curved lines.

The second type of flowmeter and the most commonly used by anaesthetists is not based upon a fixed resistance but upon a fixed pressure difference whose resistance varies with flow, the *rotameter*. It consists of a light weight bobbin in an accurately tapered glass tube such as that shown in Figure 58. The bore of the vertical glass tube increases from below upwards, so that as the bobbin is carried higher by the stream of gas, the annular space between the bobbin and the glass tube increases. The meter has a constant pressure difference across the bobbin, proportional to its weight. As flow changes the bobbin moves up and down the tube, thereby varying the annular space and hence the resistance to flow so as to always maintain the same pressure difference across the bobbin. In order to stabilize the bobbin in the centre of the tube, it is fluted so as to make it spin. The vertical tube is marked with a scale showing the height to which the bobbin will rise for a given flow.

The annular space between the bobbin and the tube wall is wide at high flows, and narrow at low flows (see Figure 58). The

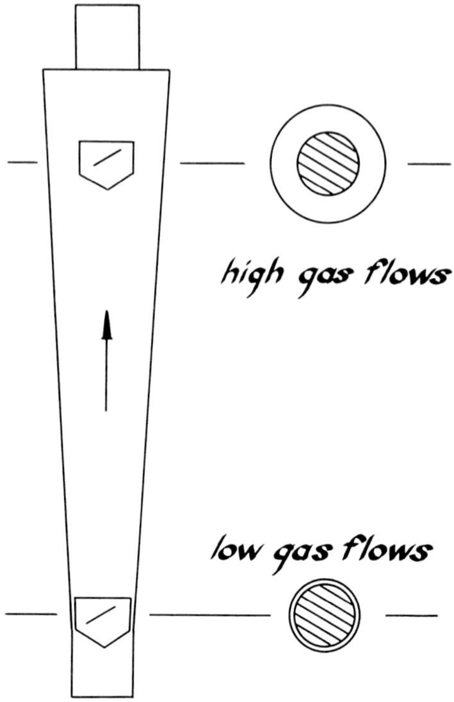

Figure 58. Rotameter.

constriction offered to the flow thereby tends to be orifice-like at high flows, and like a narrow tube at low flows. The resistance is, therefore, a laminar flow resistance at low flows, and a turbulent resistance at high flows, so that both the viscosity and the density of the gas affect the calibration of the rotameter. Rotameters must be calibrated and used for one specific gas only. Note also that viscosity and density are temperature and pressure dependent so that the calibration only applies accurately for a specified temperature and pressure.

PROBLEM 10

(a) Air flows through one inch internal diameter tubing at a peak flow of 25 l/min. during spontaneous respiration. Assuming incompressible flow (ρ constant) and a horizontal tube; is the flow laminar or turbulent? Does this tubing constitute a resistance load for the patient? What is the pressure loss in cm H_2O of a 2 metre length?

(b) A transfusion set is in use but the flow is half that required. What change would you make to double the flow by altering: a) the needle bore; b) the height of the bag? What assumption are you making for these calculations?

Chapter 11

ELECTRICITY

ELECTRICAL AND ELECTRONIC devices form an increasing part of anaesthetic procedures, particularly in the role of patient monitoring. While the anaesthetist need not understand the operation of such devices in detail, it is, nevertheless, essential to understand some basic principles of electricity in order to use them intelligently; to know their limitations and possible errors. Since the subject of electricity forms a whole branch of engineering, it is not surprising that only a few selected concepts may be presented in this chapter.

CHARGE, VOLTAGE AND CURRENT

From the atomic theory of Chapter 5, recall that electrons are negatively charged, while the protons in the atomic nucleus are positively charged. An atom with an equal number of protons and electrons is, therefore, neutral with respect to its external environment, but an atom possessing an excess of electrons is negatively charged (a negative ion), and an atom with a deficit of electrons is positively charged (a positive ion). In liquids, ions are free to move, and they constitute mobile charge carriers, but in solids, the atoms are locked into a lattice structure. However, the very energy relationships that bond the atoms of the lattice structure may provide electrons with sufficient energy to move freely within the lattice structure, and these constitute the mobile charge carriers of solids. Materials that permit the free movement of electrons (mostly metals) are called *conductors*, and those that do not are called nonconductors or *insulators*. An important group of solid materials with properties between these two extremes are called *semiconductors*, in which charge may be carried by mobile electrons (negative), or by mobile positive "holes" (electrons missing from the atomic lattice structure).

This chapter will consider some elementary rules that govern the conduction of charge in materials by electrons. Simplistically, we can therefore define a *negative charge* as an excess of electrons and a *positive charge* as a deficit of electrons. It is evident from this definition that equal negative and positive charges cancel to neutrality when they meet, and also that negative charges attract positive charges. Charge is usually given the symbol Q in electrical engineering and is measured in coulombs (C), an S.I. unit named after Charles Augustin Coulomb (1736-1806), the French physicist.

In order to produce a negative charge, electrons must be moved, leaving behind an equal positive charge. Because the charges attract one another, work must be done to produce the separation, and so the charges must gain a potential energy equal to the work done on them. This P.E. gained by the positive and negative charges is called a *potential difference* between the two charges. A potential difference (symbols E and V) also exists between any charge and neutrality, or between unequal charges. The more positive the charge, the higher is the potential difference with respect to neutrality. The S.I. unit of potential difference is the volt (symbol V), named in honour of Count Allessandro Volta (1745-1827), the Italian physicist. Potential difference is defined by the equation

$$E = \frac{W}{Q},$$

where:

E = the potential difference in volts,
W = the energy expended in separating the charges in joules,

and

Q = the electrical charge in coulombs.

The term *voltage* is often used, rather loosely, to refer to potential difference. For example, voltage might refer to the potential difference of some point with respect to neutrality. If the charge is positive the voltage is positive, but if the charge is negative then the voltage is negative. The potential difference between one point and another might be referred to as a voltage difference, a voltage drop or simply a voltage.

Neutrality, which could also be thought of as zero potential difference or zero voltage, is often labelled as *earth* or *ground.* This practice arises from the use of the earth's crust as an infinite reservoir for both types of charge. A connection to earth or ground is considered to be capable of accepting or supplying any amount of either type of charge.

Just as a fluid flows from high pressure to low pressure, and heat flows from high temperature to low temperature, electric charge thus flows from high voltage to low voltage. The flow of electric charge is called a *current* (symbol I) and is measured in amperes (symbol A), an S.I. unit named after André-Marie Ampere (1775-1836), the French physicist. One ampere is defined as the steady flow of one coulomb of charge per second;

$$I = \frac{dQ}{dt},$$

instantaneously,
or in the averaged case,

$$I = \frac{Q}{t},$$

where:

I = current in amperes (A),
Q = charge in coulombs,
t = time in seconds.

Analogies are often drawn between electricity and fluids, and can be useful because some of the concepts developed in electrical engineering may be analogously transferred to fluid mechanics. Anaesthetists especially may find it useful to use their understanding of fluid mechanics as an aid to understanding electrical concepts. Fluid volume is analogous to charge, current is analogous to fluid flow, and pressure is analogous to potential difference (voltage).

RESISTANCE

As mobile charge carriers flow through a material they continually buffet the molecular structure and thereby lose (transfer) their K.E. This loss of energy is in the form of heat and is unrecoverable; it may thus be thought of as due to an electrical friction or resistance to current flow. The energy loss due to resistance causes a potential difference to be developed along the current path, and this loss of voltage is called a voltage drop. The electrical situation is analogous to the fluid mechanical situation in which the flow of fluid through a flow resistance incurs a drop in pressure.

George Simon Ohm (1787-1854), the German physicist, discovered that the ratio of the potential difference (voltage) between two points in a material, and the current flowing through it, was a constant for most materials; the *resistance* (symbol R) of the material. Symbolically, Ohm's law is:

$$R = \frac{E}{I},$$

where:

R = the resistance of the material in ohms (symbol Ω),
E = the potential difference in volts,

and

I = the current in amperes.

It is customary to conceptualize resistance as a localized (lumped) property even though it is distributed throughout a material. In electric circuits, resistance is usually considered to be confined to discrete devices called *resistors* which are designed to exhibit specific values of resistance. The wires connecting resistors to different parts of the circuit are made of low resistance material (copper) and are usually considered to possess negligible resistance.

Examine the electric circuit shown in Figure 59. It uses standard symbols to show a battery connected to a resistor by copper

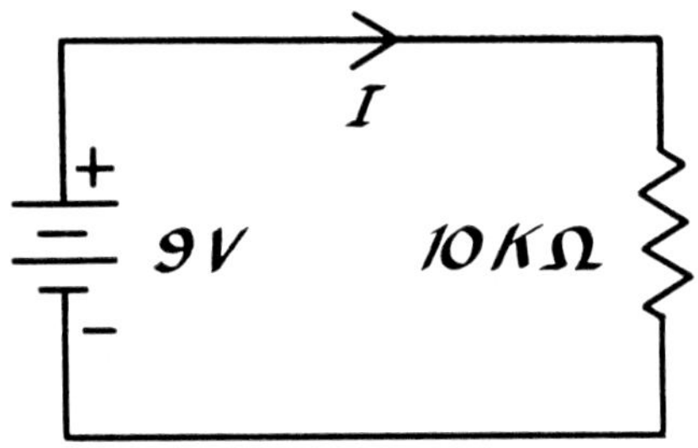

Figure 59. Simple electric circuit.

wire so as to form an electric circuit. The *battery* is assumed to be an ideal device which maintains a constant potential difference (in this case 9 V) between its terminals (one positive and the other negative) and is capable of supplying any current. The battery is, therefore, analogous to a constant pressure ventilator (on continuous inspiration). Because of the circuit connections, the battery voltage is applied to the resistor, and as a result, a current flows through the resistor. According to Ohm's law,

$$R = \frac{E}{I},$$

and therefore,

$$I = \frac{E}{R} = \frac{9\ \text{V}}{10\text{k}\Omega} = 0.9\ \text{mA}.$$

The resistor dissipates energy supplied from the battery as unrecoverable heat. The rate of energy dissipation can be calculated as follows:
By definition,

$$E = \frac{W}{Q},$$

and also by definition,

$$Q = It.$$

Therefore,

$$W = EQ = EIt,$$

and

$$\frac{W}{t} = EI.$$

We recognize W/t as the rate of energy dissipation, that is power P. The resistor, therefore, dissipates energy at the rate of,

$$P = EI \quad \text{watts (W)},$$

or using Ohm's law,

$$P = I^2R = \frac{E^2}{R}\ \text{watts.}$$

In the circuit of Figure 59,

$$P = EI = 9 \times 0.9 \times 10^{-3} = 8.1\ \text{mW}.$$

This simple circuit illustrates a law which is used to analyze much more complicated circuits; the battery, as a source of elec-

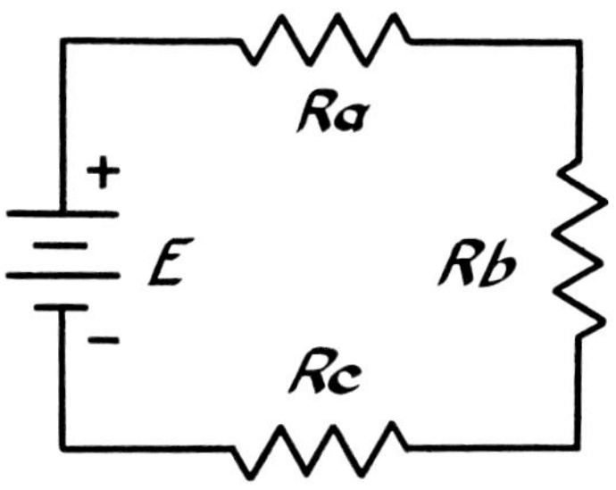

Figure 60. Series electric circuit.

trical energy, is called a *voltage rise,* in the direction of the current flow. The resistor, as a dissipator of electrical energy, is called a *voltage drop.* The law is named after Gustav Robert Kirchoff (1824-1887), the German physicist. *Kirchoff's voltage law* states that around any complete circuit (in the direction of current flow) the sum of the voltage rises equals the sum of the voltage drops. In the simple circuit of Figure 59, Kirchoff's law simply states the obvious fact that the battery voltage is applied across the resistor. However, consider the series circuit shown in Figure 60.

A battery of voltage E is applied to a circuit containing three resistors in series. The voltage drops across each resistor are Ea, Eb, Ec respectively. For each coulomb of charge, Q, the amount of energy lost in the resistors is

$$\frac{Wa}{Q} + \frac{Wb}{Q} + \frac{Wc}{Q}.$$

This energy loss is equal to the energy gain provided by the battery, that is

$$\frac{W}{Q}.$$

So,

$$\frac{W}{Q} = \frac{Wa}{Q} + \frac{Wb}{Q} + \frac{Wc}{Q}.$$

But

$$\frac{W}{Q} = E, \quad \frac{Wa}{Q} = Ea, \quad \frac{Wb}{Q} = Eb,$$

and

$$\frac{Wc}{Q} = Ec.$$

Therefore, $E = Ea + Eb + Ec$, which is a symbolic statement of Kirchoff's voltage law.

If we wished to replace the three resistors in the series circuit by a single resistor which would have an equivalent effect, we could find the value of the equivalent resistance, *Re*, as follows:

Since

$$E = Ea + Eb + Ec,$$

and since

$$Ea = IRa,\ Eb = IRb,\ Ec = IRc,$$

because current *I* flows through all three resistors, therefore,

$$E = IRa + IRb + IRc,$$

and

$$E = I(Ra + Rb + Rc).$$

The equivalent resistance is thus,

$$Re = Ra + Rb + Rc.$$

For resistors in parallel circuits, such as that shown in Figure 61, the equivalent resistance can be shown to be

$$Re = \frac{1}{\frac{1}{Ra} + \frac{1}{Rb} + \frac{1}{Rc}},$$

and for the special case of two resistors in parallel:

$$Re = \frac{R_1R_2}{R_1 + R_2}.$$

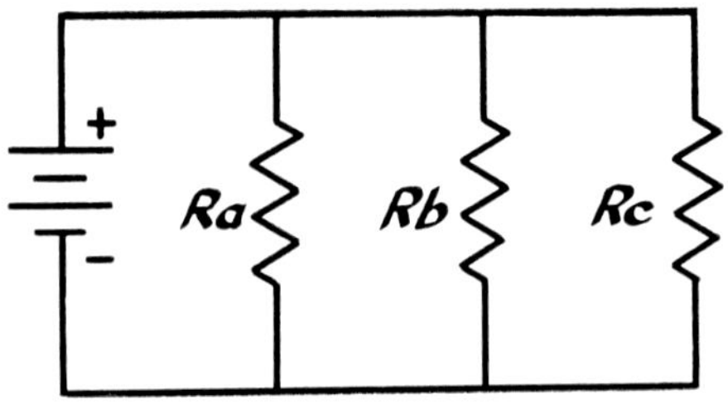

Figure 61. Parallel electric circuit.

It should be noted that these laws of the series and parallel circuits apply by analogy to series and parallel laminar flow resistances.

CAPACITANCE

A *capacitor* is an electrical device for storing charge. It consists of two parallel plates or sheets of conductor separated by a thin layer of nonconducting material called the *dielectric*. When a battery is connected to the plates of a capacitor (shown schematically in Figure 62) it fills one plate of the capacitor (condenser) with positive charge and the other plate with negative charge. The charges cannot cancel each other because the dielectric prevents them from coming into contact. Once the plates have filled with charge, so that the potential difference between the two plates is equal and opposite in polarity to the battery voltage, then the current flow from the battery stops.

An *electric field* exists between the plates of the charged capacitor due to the attraction between charges of opposite polarity. We could detect the presence of the electric field by observing that a mobile charge within that space between the plates would be accelerated by a force toward the plate of the opposite polarity. Because the establishment of this electric field required energy from the battery in order to crowd together like charges, which repel each other, onto each plate, we think of the initial charging of a capacitor as the storing of energy in the form of an electric field within the dielectric.

When the battery is disconnected from the capacitor it leaves the capacitor charged, with a voltage (potential difference) between its plates equal to that of the battery. If a resistor is now

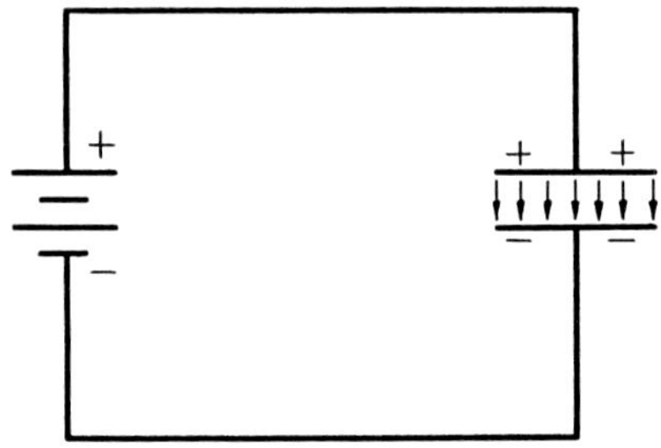

Figure 62. Capacitor connected to a battery.

connected to the capacitor, current will be pushed off the plates by the capacitor voltage which declines as the charge decreases. The energy which was stored in the electric field is returned to the circuit and dissipated in the resistor as the field and capacitor voltage decline.

A capacitor stores an amount of charge, Q, which depends upon the geometry of the device and the voltage, V, applied across the plates. The *capacitance,* C, of a particular capacitor is defined as the constant of proportionality between Q and V, that is

$$Q = CV,$$

and

$$C = \frac{Q}{V}$$

where:

C = capacitance in farads,
Q = charge in coulombs,
V = potential difference between the plates in volts.

The farad (symbol F) is the S.I. unit of capacitance and was named for Michael Faraday (1791-1867), the English physicist and chemist.

Capacitance is the electrical analogue of compliance. Instead of storing a volume of gas for a given applied pressure, a capacitor stores an amount of charge for a given applied voltage.

The process of charging a capacitance through a resistance is directly analogous to that of filling a compliance through a flow resistance by the application of a positive pressure. Figure 63 details the electric circuit, the differential equation governing the process, and the graphical solution, all of which may be taken by analogy from the development in Chapter 2.

At time zero switch 1 is closed and switch 2 left open. Current flow starts at a value $I = V/R$ and falls exponentially to zero with a time constant RC. The voltage across the capacitor starts at zero and rises exponentially to a value equal to the battery voltage with a time constant RC. The steady state current is zero, and the voltage across the capacitor equals the battery voltage but with an opposing polarity.

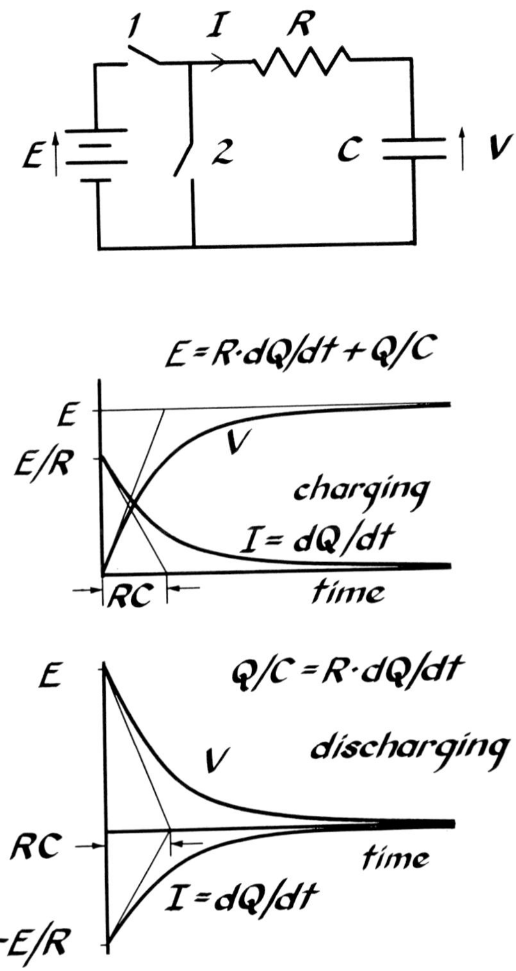

Figure 63. Charging and discharging of a capacitor through a resistor.

The discharge of the capacitor through the resistor (switch 1 open, switch 2 closed at time zero), also shown in Figure 63, is analogous to passive expiration. The time constant for the exponential decay of V is again RC. The current flow is in the opposite direction to the charging current because the voltage across the capacitor opposes the battery voltage.

Capacitors, like resistors, may be combined in series and parallel circuit arrangements, and the formulas for finding the single equivalent capacitance are as follows:

For parallel capacitors:

$$Ce = C_1 + C_2 + C_3 + \ldots\ldots$$

For series capacitors:

$$\frac{1}{Ce} = \frac{1}{C_1} + \frac{1}{C_2} + \frac{1}{C_3} + \ldots\ldots$$

Note that these two formulas are the reverse of those for resistors.

INDUCTANCE

When a battery is first connected to the ends of a long length of copper wire, the current rises quickly, but not instantaneously, to a value determined by Ohm's law. However, if the same length of wire is wound into a coil and then connected to the battery, the current rises more slowly; and, if an iron core is inserted into the coil and the connection repeated, then the current rises even more slowly. It is customary to think of the cause for this sluggishness or lagging of the current as being due to a counter or back voltage opposing that of the battery. But what causes the back voltage? To answer this question we must digress slightly into electromagnetism.

Moving charges (current) gives rise to a phenomenon called a *magnetic field.* Figure 64 shows how the magnetic field vectors (flux) around a single wire carrying current can be concentrated by coiling the wire into a helix and then further concentrated by providing an iron core for the helix (a magnetic field passes through iron more easily than air). The magnetic flux lines are shown as vectors in Figure 64 with a characteristic direction determined by the direction of the current.

Magnetic fields like that in the iron core can be permanently induced in special materials, and the end at which the flux leaves the material is called the *north pole* while the end at which the flux enters is called *south pole.* The north and south nomenclature is derived from the function of the first useful magnet, the compass needle. Experiments with magnets show that an attrac-

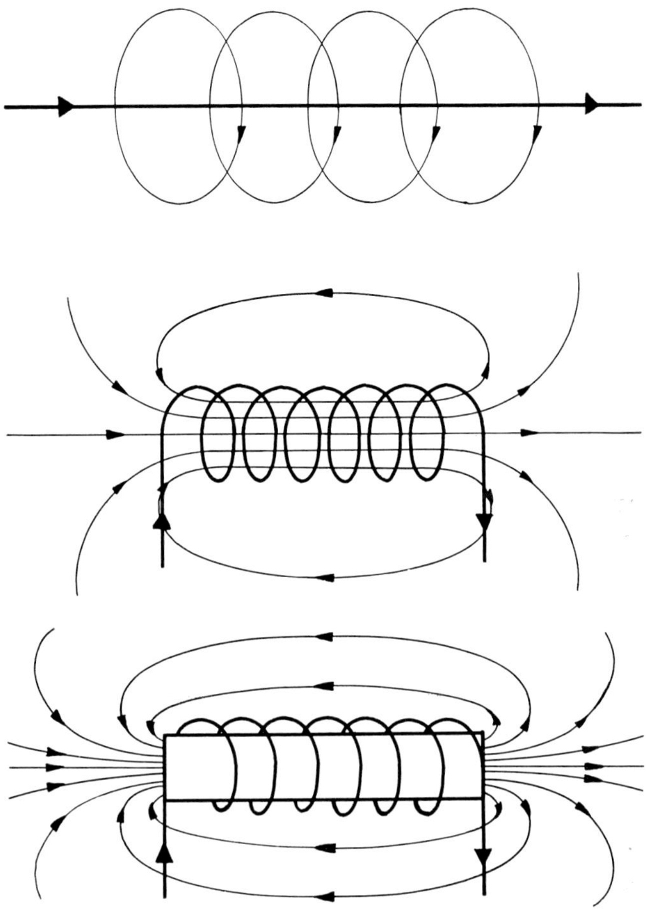

Figure 64. Magnetic field produced by electric current.

tive force exists between magnetic poles of opposite types while like magnetic poles repel.

Michael Faraday studied the movement of a wire through a magnetic field and found that a voltage was induced in the wire that was proportional to the rate at which the wire encountered the magnetic field. He also noted that the induced voltage was such that its polarity would produce a current in the wire which, in turn, would produce a magnetic field around the wire whose magnetic force lines were directed so as to repel the standing magnetic field. The repelling force meant that a force was required to move the wire through the field. Figure 65 shows a commonly used demonstration of *Faraday's law.* It shows a wire forced through a magnetic field with velocity v. The result of this movement is a voltage induced in the wire which produces current I with its attendant magnetic field. Although not shown, the reverse causal sequence is also possible. A wire carrying a current I in a magnetic field would experience a force which would tend to move it in the opposite direction to that pictured in Figure 65. These paired phenomena are the principles which underlie electric generators and motors respectively.

Returning to the original question of what causes the back voltage in the wire, we can now say that this voltage is induced in the wire by the growing magnetic field caused by the increasing current through the wire. As the current increases so does the accompanying magnetic field. Its increasing strength causes it to

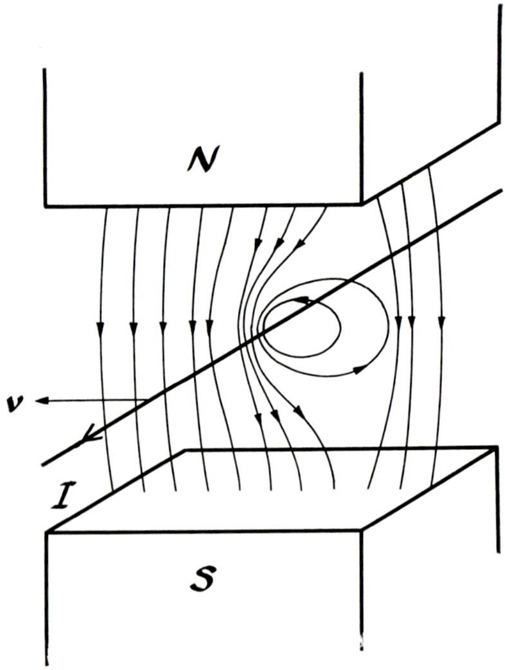

Figure 65. Demonstration of Faraday's law.

expand, i.e. the force lines move outwards, thereby cutting through the wire as if the wire were moving through a stationary magnetic field and inducing the back voltage. The coiling of the wire and the insertion of an iron core into the coil both serve to concentrate the magnetic field and strengthen the effect. Ultimately then, it is the current itself that is responsible for its own sluggishness, and the phenomenon is called *self-induction.*

Once the current reaches its steady state value determined by Ohm's law, the magnetic field is constant; magnetic force lines no longer move through the conducting wire, and the back voltage is zero. The energy drawn from the battery to establish the current is now stored in the magnetic field. Should the battery now be removed and a resistor substituted, the current will decrease as the resistor dissipates energy. Its fall is delayed, however, because the decreasing magnetic field now induces a voltage directed so as to maintain the current. The polarity of the back voltage is reversed because the magnetic field lines are collapsing and moving in the opposite direction to that during build-up. The energy expended by the back voltage in slowing the current decrease is equal to that stored in the magnetic field. Thus, any conductor carrying a current stores energy in a magnetic field while current is increasing, and gets it back when current is decreasing. The effect is enhanced by coiling the wire and by providing an iron core. A device designed to exhibit this property is called an *inductor,* and it possesses the characteristic called *inductance.*

Heinrich Friedrich Emil Lenz (1809-1865), the German physicist, noted that in any inductor there is a proportionality between the back voltage and the rate of change of current. The proportionality constant, which depends upon the geometry and materials of the inductor is called the inductance, and given the symbol L. The S.I. unit of inductance is the henry, symbol H, named after Joseph Henry (1797-1878), the American physicist.

Lenz's law

$$V_L \propto -\frac{dI}{dt},$$

and

$$V_L = -L\frac{dI}{dt},$$

where:

L = the inductance in henrys,
V_L = the back voltage in volts,
I = the current in amperes.

The negative sign indicates that V_L and dI/dt are in the opposite direction, that is V_L opposes the direction of change of I.

It is interesting to rearrange this equation slightly and compare it to a familiar mechanics equation:

$$V_L = -L\frac{dI}{dt}.$$

Recall that

$$I = \frac{dQ}{dt}.$$

Therefore

$$\frac{dI}{dt} = \frac{d^2Q}{dt^2},$$

the second derivative of charge with respect to time, that is the acceleration of charge.

Now compare

$$-V_L = L\frac{d^2Q}{dt^2},$$

with

$$F = Ma.$$

The comparison shows that inductance is the electrical analogue of mass and may be thought of as giving rise to electrical inertia.

Consider the circuit shown in Figure 66. When switch 1 is closed and switch 2 open, the equation relating the magnitudes of V and the current I is

$$V = L\frac{dI}{dt}.$$

This differential equation solves to show that the current starts at zero and rises exponentially to a steady value $I = E/R$ with a time constant L/R. The back voltage V starts at a value equal and opposite to the battery voltage E, and decays to zero exponentially with a time constant L/R.

When switch 1 is opened and switch 2 closed, the back voltage

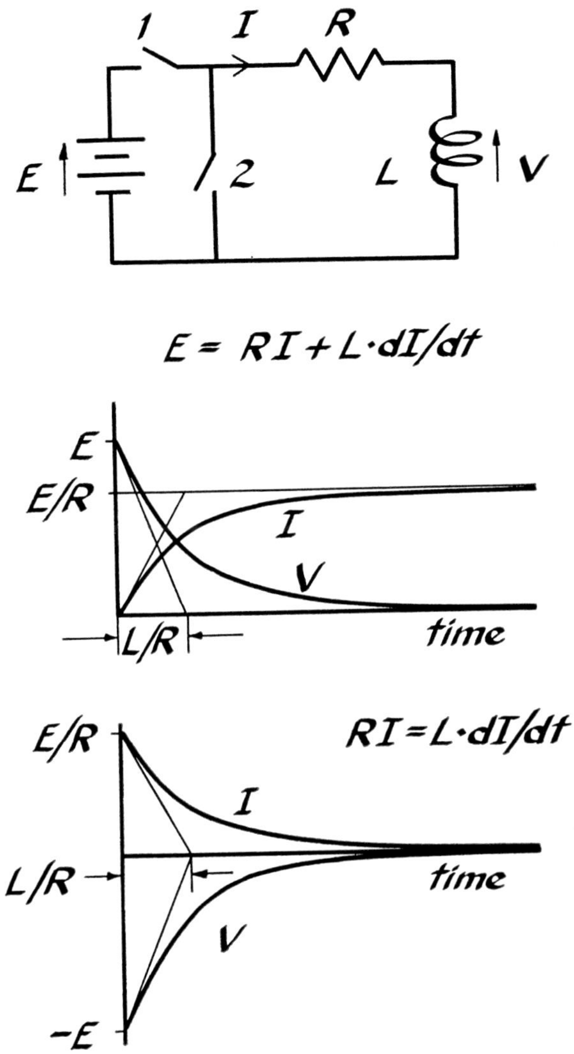

Figure 66. Plot of voltage and current versus time for a series circuit of an inductor and a resistor connected to a battery, upper plot, and then to a conductor, lower plot.

polarity is reversed so that it attempts to maintain the current. Current decays exponentially from a value $I = E/R$ to zero with a time constant L/R. The back voltage is reversed and equals E initially but decays exponentially to zero with a time constant L/R.

THE ELECTROMAGNETIC FLOWMETER

Having introduced Faraday's law in this section it is appropriate to digress slightly and consider an application of this law, which is of interest to anaesthetists. Figure 67 shows a sketch illustrating the principle of the electromagnetic flowmeter. A magnetic field is applied across an exposed blood vessel so that the blood flows through the field at right angles to it. Because blood is a conductor moving through a magnetic field, Faraday's law says that a voltage should be generated at the walls of the vessel at points mutually perpendicular to both the magnetic field and the flow direction. Electrodes placed against the outer wall of the vessel can pick-up this voltage which is proportional to both the magnetic field strength and the flow velocity. In this way a signal proportional to flow may be obtained. In practice the magnetic field is provided by an electromagnet (coil plus iron core)

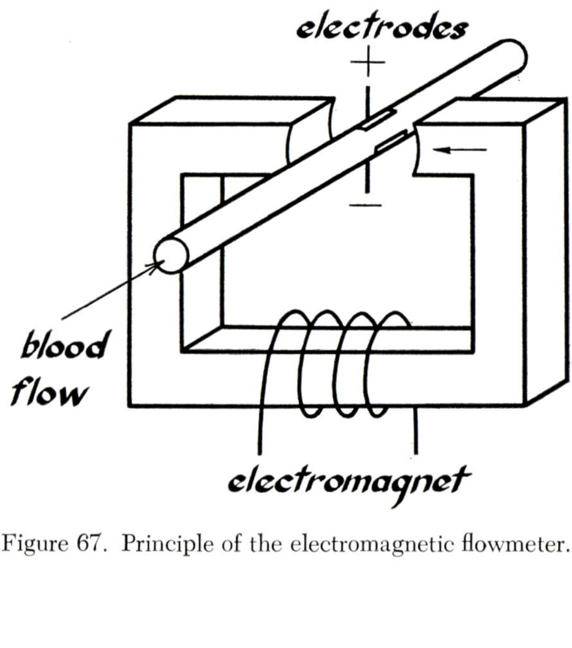

Figure 67. Principle of the electromagnetic flowmeter.

whose magnetic field polarity alternates in either a sine wave or square wave pattern so as to avoid problems with electrode polarization.

PROBLEM 11

(a) Develop the formula for the equivalent resistance of two resistors in parallel,

$$Re = \frac{R_1 R_2}{R_1 + R_2},$$

from first principles. If R_1 and R_2 are 100Ω each and are connected to a 12V battery, at what rate is energy dissipated in each resistor? Note that commercially produced resistors have power ratings according to the energy dissipation they can handle safely: ¼W, ½W, 1W, 5W, etc.

(b) A relay is an electric switch operated by an electromagnet. When the current of the electromagnet is turned on, the magnetic field builds up until it is strong enough to attract an iron lever which operates the electric switch. Relays are designed so that control currents of a few milliamperes can energize the electromagnet and operate an electric relay switch which controls currents of many amperes. In this way, a small current switch can control very large currents. The electromagnetic circuit is similar to that of Figure 66 with switch 1 as the control switch.

A battery of 12 volts was used to operate a relay coil (electromagnet) whose inductance was 60 mH and whose resistance was 100Ω. The relay switch operated when the current in the coil reached 0.114A. How long was the time delay between the operation of the control switch and the operation of the relay switch?

Chapter 12

A.C. CIRCUITS

A.C. AND D.C. CIRCUITS

THE PRECEDING CHAPTER introduced the elements of resistance, capacitance and inductance. So far we have examined their behaviour when connected to batteries, sources of current at a steady voltage. In these circuits, after the initial transient changes, the currents and voltages reach a steady state or level. Such a circuit is called a direct current (D.C.) circuit. As well as standing for direct current, the term D.C. has also become synonymous with steady, unchanging voltages and currents, which maintain nonzero values over periods of time.

The contrasting companion of the D.C. circuit is the alternating current (A.C.) circuit, in which voltages and currents fluctuate above and below zero (positive and negative) continually. The typical waveform of the A.C. circuit is the sine wave, continuously varying positive and negative in a smooth symmetrical time course.

Some circuits have voltages and currents which may be classified as both A.C. and D.C. Consider the electrical signal from a pressure transducer which replicates blood pressure. The electrical signal is thought of as consisting of the sum of a D.C. component, corresponding to the steady mean pressure, and an A.C. component, corresponding to the pulse pressure variation above and below the mean pressure.

THE ROTATING VECTOR CONCEPT

Before examining the behaviour of resistors, inductors and capacitors in A.C. circuits, it is necessary to review the sine wave considered in Chapter 1 and introduce the rotating vector representation of sine waves. The sine wave variation of a voltage, V, for example, is described by the following equation:

$$V = Vm \sin(2\pi ft),$$

where:

V = the voltage at any time,
Vm = the maximum voltage (+ or −), the amplitude,
f = the frequency of the sine wave in Hz,

and

t = the time in seconds.

Since the sine wave is generated geometrically by a point on the periphery of a rotating wheel, voltage V can therefore be represented by a *rotating vector,* such as is shown in Figure 68. The frequency of the sine wave $(1/T)$ is represented by the angular rotation of the vector at a speed of $2\pi f$ radians per second, and the amplitude of the sine wave is represented by the length of the vector, equal to Vm, half the peak-to-peak value.

The rotating vector concept of the sine wave is extremely useful in displaying the differences in timing between two sine waves of the same frequency. Figure 69 shows two sine waves: one for voltage V and the other for current I. The current variation occurs a little later in time than that of voltage. On the rotating vector plot, this time difference is indicated by an angle ϕ called the *phase angle* between the voltage and current. The situation would be described by saying that current lags voltage by

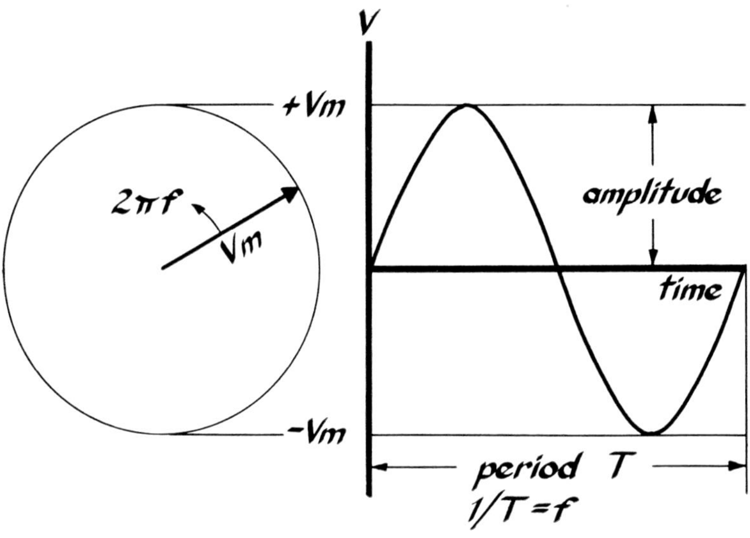

Figure 68. Rotating vector representation of a sine wave.

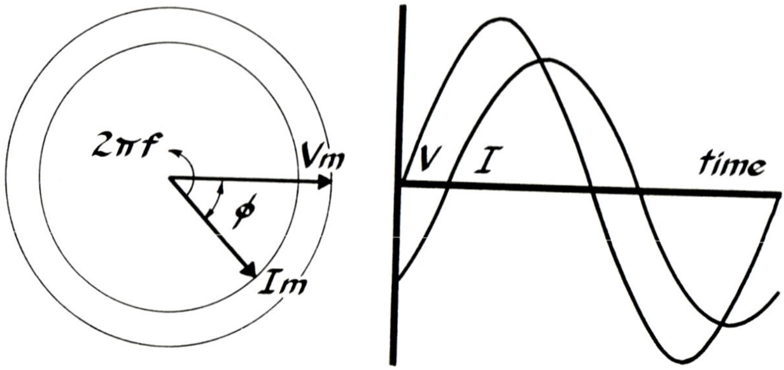

Figure 69. Concept of phase difference.

a phase angle ϕ or that voltage leads current by a phase angle ϕ. When there is no delay between sine waves and the phase angle is zero, then the sine waves would be said to be *in phase* with each other.

A.C. AND RESISTANCE

Examine the electric circuit shown in Figure 70. It uses standard symbols to show an A.C. generator connected to a resistance. The A.C. generator is assumed to be an ideal device which

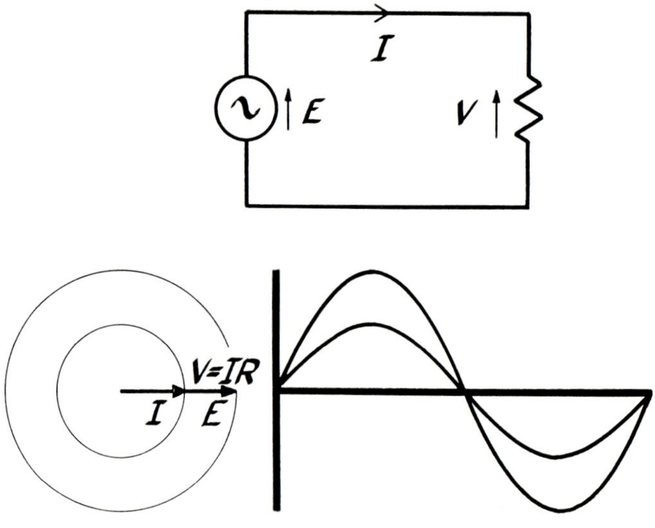

Figure 70. A.C. and resistance.

maintains a sine wave potential difference, E, of constant amplitude between its terminals and is capable of supplying any current. The arrow associated with the generator arbitrarily indicates that the top terminal is positive with respect to the bottom terminal when the sine wave E is positive. Similarly the current I and voltage V arrows designate the positive direction of the sine waves. It is customary to use directions which would be found in a D.C. circuit so that when E goes positive I will flow in the designated direction, and V will be positive in the direction of the arrow so as to resist the current.

Kirchoff's law applies to this circuit, and

$$V = E.$$

Ohm's law also applies to this circuit, and

$$V = IR \text{ or } I = V/R.$$

The dissipation of energy by a resistance in an A.C. circuit is calculated somewhat differently than that in a D.C. circuit. While it is true that the instantaneous rate of energy loss is

$$P = VI,$$

where:

$$V = Vm \sin(2\pi ft),$$

and

$$I = Im \sin(2\pi ft),$$

this is not the average rate of dissipation. To find the average power it is necessary to integrate the instantaneous power over a complete cycle. When this integration is performed it is found that

$$P(\text{avg.}) = \frac{Vm}{\sqrt{2}} \times \frac{Im}{\sqrt{2}},$$

or

$$P = Ve \cdot Ie = Ie^2 \cdot R = Ve^2/R,$$

where:

$$Ve = Vm/\sqrt{2} = 0.707\ Vm,$$

and

$$Ie = Im/\sqrt{2} = 0.707\ Im.$$

Ve and *Ie* are called the *effective* values of voltage and current. They are also known as the *root-mean-square* (rms) values.

In addition to being useful in power calculations, effective values are those read by moving-coil meters because of their integrative effect. Because the effective values can be used in both Ohm's law and power calculation and are also the values measured by A.C. meters, they are used almost exclusively in A.C., sine wave circuits. Unless otherwise specified, voltages and currents in A.C. circuits can be assumed to be expressed as effective values. This use also applies to rotating vector and sine wave diagrams where effective values are used in place of maximum values.

A.C. AND INDUCTANCE

When a sine wave of voltage, *V*, is applied to a pure inductance (zero resistance), it will produce a sine wave of current, *I*, through the inductance, *L*. Energy is stored in the magnetic field as current increases and is returned when current decreases. Over a complete cycle, the energy dissipation for an inductance is, therefore, zero.

The back voltage across the inductance, V_L, is equal and opposite in polarity to the driving voltage, *V*, as shown in the cir-

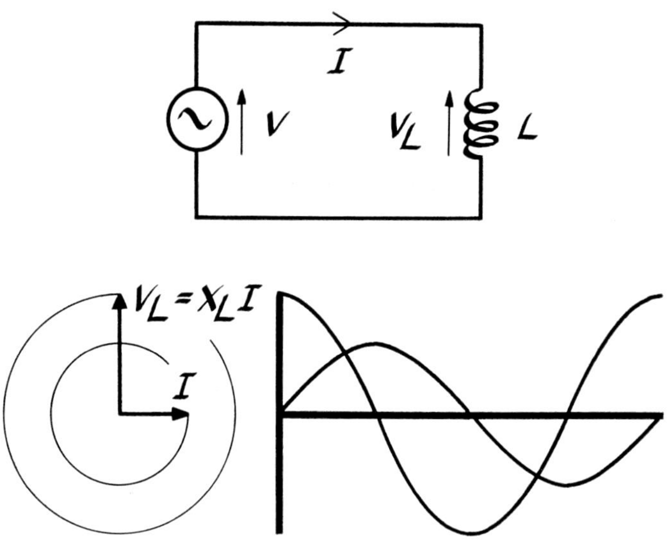

Figure 71. A.C. and inductance.

cuit diagram of Figure 71. The back voltage and the current are related by Lenz's law; therefore,

$$V = -L \frac{dI}{dt} = -V_L.$$

The negative sign indicates an opposing polarity.

We can assume that current is sinusoidal so, since,

$$I = Im \cdot \sin (2\pi ft),$$

therefore,

$$V_L = L \cdot Im \cdot \frac{d\sin (2\pi ft)}{dt}.$$

The differentiation formula for a sine function is

$$\frac{d\sin (2\pi ft)}{dt} = 2\pi f \cdot \cos(2\pi ft),$$

so,

$$V_L = L \cdot Im \cdot 2\pi f \cdot \cos (2\pi ft).$$

But trigonometrically,

$$\cos \theta = \sin (\theta + 90°);$$

that is, a sine wave advanced by 90° becomes a cosine wave. Therefore

$$V_L = 2\pi fL \cdot Im \cdot \sin (2\pi ft + 90°).$$

The equation states that in a pure inductance circuit, the current lags behind the voltage across the inductance, V_L, by 90 degrees. The rotating vector diagram and resulting waveforms are shown in Figure 71. One way to conceptualize the reason for the lagging current is to visualize the build up of the magnetic field as causing a retardation of the current by inducing a back voltage. As a result, current reaches any given value later than it would have reached that value if the induced back voltage were absent.

In the above equation, the magnitudes of the rotating vectors are related by the constants $2\pi fL$. Because an inductance does not resist the passage of a current like a resistance but does react against its passage by producing a back voltage it is said to possess a characteristic called *inductive reactance* instead of resistance. Inductive reactance is given the symbol X_L and defined as

$$X_L = 2\pi f L \quad \text{(ohms)},$$

so that it can be used in an Ohm's law for the inductance:

$$V_L = X_L \cdot I \text{ or } I = V_L / X_L,$$

which results from the phase relation equation derived from Lenz's law. Unlike the phase relation equation, Ohm's law for the inductance relates magnitudes only.

Inductive reactance, unlike resistance, is dependent upon frequency; the higher the frequency, the greater the reactance. An inductance therefore allows D.C. to pass easily but progressively opposes A.C. as frequency increases.

A.C. AND CAPACITANCE

The effect of a capacitance in an A.C. circuit on the phase relationship between current and voltage is opposite to that of an inductance. Because current must flow onto the plates of a capacitance before the voltage can build up, current leads voltage. During charge build up, energy is stored in the electric field

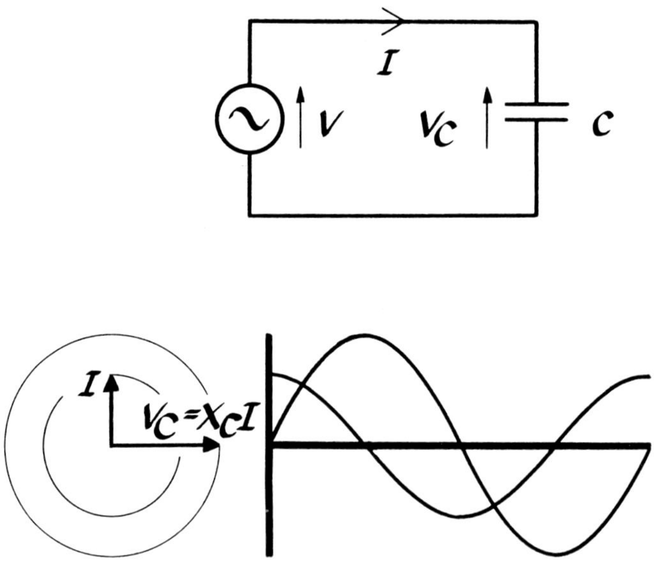

Figure 72. A.C. and capacitance.

within the dielectric, but as current flow reverses and voltage declines, the electric field collapses yielding its stored energy, so that over the complete cycle of a sine wave the energy consumed by a capacitance is zero.

The voltage across a pure capacitance (zero resistance), *Vc,* is equal and opposite in polarity to the driving voltage, *V*, as shown in the circuit diagram in Figure 72. *Vc* and *I* are related by the following equation.

$$I = C \frac{dVc}{dt}$$

Since

$$Vc = Vcm \cdot \sin (2\pi ft)$$

$$I = C \cdot Vcm \cdot \frac{d\sin (2\pi ft)}{dt}$$

and

$$I = 2\pi fC \cdot Vcm \cdot \cos (2\pi ft)$$

But trigonometrically,

$$\cos \theta = \sin (\theta + 90°),$$

therefore,

$$I = 2\pi fC \cdot Vcm \cdot \sin (2\pi ft + 90°).$$

The equation states that in a pure capacitance circuit, the current leads the voltage across the capacitance, *Vc,* by 90°. The rotating vector diagram and resulting waveforms are shown in Figure 72.

From the D.C. analysis of the capacitance we know that current cannot pass through a capacitance because of the dielectric separating the plates. In an A.C. circuit this is true as well, but because the charge alternately flows on and off both plates, the capacitance appears to pass an A.C. current, and an A.C. meter in the circuit would indicate that the capacitance was conducting current.

For this reason, Ohm's law may be applied to the capacitance just as it was applied to the inductance. The quantity relating current and voltage is termed *capacitive reactance* (symbol *Xc*), and its value from the phase relation equation is

$$Xc = \frac{1}{2\pi fC}.$$

Ohm's law for capacitance is

$$Vc = Xc \cdot I \text{ or } I = Vc/Xc.$$

Again, note that this equation relates magnitudes only and does not show the phase relation of Vc and I.

Capacitive reactance, like inductive reactance, is dependent upon frequency, but contrastingly, it is inversely dependent; the higher the frequency, the smaller the reactance. A capacitance, therefore, blocks D.C. but progressively allows A.C. to pass more easily as frequency increases.

IMPEDANCE

So far we have considered single elements in A.C. circuits. When more than one element is included, the situation becomes more complex. The methods and mathematics are more complicated than those used so far and knowledge of them is not justified for anaesthetists. However, the term *impedance* is encountered by anaesthetists, and, although it need not be fully understood, the anaesthetist should know enough about impedance so as not to treat it as resistance.

Consider the series *RL* circuit shown in Figure 73. The current I flows through both circuit elements and is represented by a horizontal vector on the rotating vector diagram. V_R is in phase with I and equal to IR according to Ohm's law. V_R is, therefore, also a horizontal vector on the rotating vector diagram. From our examination of the inductance we know that V_L is a vector which leads the current vector by 90°, and is equal in magnitude to $X_L I$.

Now according to Kirchoff's voltage law, the generator voltage V must equal the sum of the voltage drops $V_R + V_L$. The summation is a vector addition and is shown in Figure 73. We can think of the series R and L elements as a single element whose characteristic is an impeding of current and call it an impedance (symbol Z) measured in ohms. Impedance is defined such that Ohm's law for the circuit may be stated as

$$V = ZI \text{ or } I = V/Z$$

However, Ohm's law deals with magnitudes only, and the phase

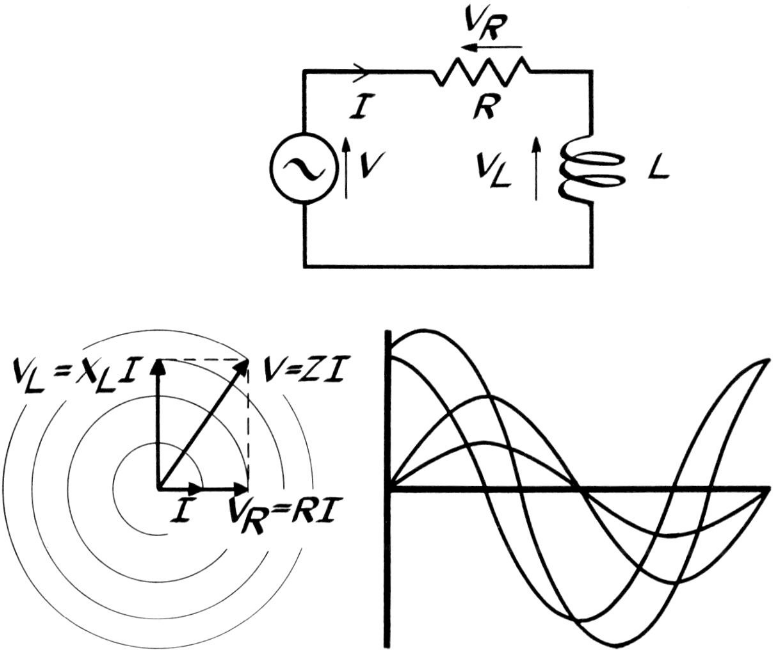

Figure 73. A.C. and inductance and resistance in series.

relationship must be determined from the rotating vector diagram. From the vector diagram, it can be seen that

$$Z = \sqrt{R^2 + X_L^2} \qquad \text{(Pythagoras)},$$

and that $\tan \theta = \dfrac{X_L}{R}$.

Suffice to say that impedance is a complex parameter whose magnitude and phase angle changes with frequency.

THE TRANSFORMER

The transformer, pictured in Figure 74, is another application of Faraday's law. It consists of two coils of wire coupled by an iron core. If an A.C. generator is applied to one coil (the primary), then a continuously varying magnetic field will be produced in the iron core by the current in the primary. Since the magnetic field is continuously varying and is coupled to the other

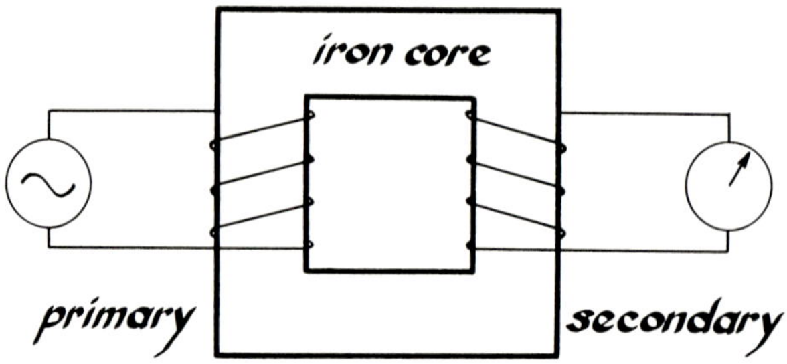

Figure 74. Transformer.

coil (the secondary) an A.C. voltage will be induced in the secondary coil.

In an ideal transformer, the coupling between primary and secondary coils is dependent upon the number of turns in each coil according to the following proportionality:

$$Vs = Vp\frac{N_2}{N_1},$$

where:

Vs = the secondary voltage,
Vp = the primary voltage,
N_1 = the number of turns in the primary coil,

and

N_2 = the number of turns in the secondary coil.

Because the secondary voltage depends upon the turns ratio, it can be made larger or smaller than the primary voltage, and this voltage changing ability is the principal use of the transformer. For example, transistorized or solid state instrumentation usually requires power voltages in the tens of volts, whereas that supplied from the mains (wall sockets) is 110/220 V A.C. A transformer is used to step-down the voltage from 110/220 to that required by the instrument electronics.

The other useful characteristic of the transformer is that, although A.C. power passes from primary to secondary circuits, D.C. does not; voltage can only be induced in the secondary by a changing magnetic field. In addition, there is no physical connection between the primary and secondary circuits; they are isolated from one another except via the magnetic induction connection. The use of a transformer as an isolation device is of interest to anaesthetists and is examined in the next section.

ELECTRIC SHOCK HAZARD

The human body is operated electro-chemically, and electric currents from external sources can disrupt this operation by overwhelming the internal control signals; cardiac muscle in particular is highly susceptible and easily fibrillates. Other muscles may also be operated improperly with resulting damage, and with high enough currents, resistive heating may cause burning, chemical breakdown and electrolysis. The data used in this chapter was taken from an article entitled "Electric Shock Hazard" by Charles F. Dalziel, in the February 1972 issue of *Spectrum* (volume 9, number 2), published by the Institute of Electrical and Electronics Engineers, Inc.

Electric shocks occur when a voltage is applied between two contacts with the body. Since the current follows a multitude of different pathways of least impedance, it is difficult to determine what route the current takes, and most electric shock data are empirical. At main power frequencies (50-60 Hz), about 80 mA causes fibrillation of the heart when the electrical contacts are applied to the skin so that the current path includes the heart (for example, right arm to left arm or right leg to left arm). Considerably less current, approximately 150 to 400 μA, is necessary if one of the electrical contacts is to a saline-filled catheter inserted into the heart. This latter shock hazard is often called *microshock*.

The impedance of the tissue pathways depends upon frequency so that the routes taken by current are different for different frequencies. Examples are: at 1 MHz several amperes may be passed between two skin electrodes (because the current does not penetrate tissues but spreads over the area of the skin), at 0 Hz, i.e. D.C., about 400 mA passed between skin electrodes causes fibrillation of the heart, and at 300 Hz microshock can require as much as 2 mA. It is unfortunate that the worst hazard occurs at frequencies which are approximately equal to those used in mains power supplies (50-60 Hz).

The basic protection from shock for the body is a high skin resistance. Dry skin has a resistance from 100 to 300 kΩ/cm² between two contacts; so that, 120 volts applied from one hand to the other through 1 cm² plates would cause about 1.2 mA to flow, not enough to cause fibrillation of the heart. However, if the skin were wet, then the skin resistance could decline to about 500Ω/cm², and then 240 mA would flow, well above the threshold for fibrillation.

Electric shock accidents have one common element: The patient becomes part of an electric circuit, with a voltage difference across the patient. In most cases, one of the two contact points is with earth/ground, that is zero voltage, and the other is with electrical apparatus where contact is made with a voltage which is not zero with respect to ground/earth. This situation applies particularly to the mains power supply; this can be seen in Figure 75; a grounded/earthed patient contacting the mains power supply experiences an electric shock because one wire of the mains supply is also grounded. The patient, therefore, becomes a conduction pathway forming a circuit with the generator. One way of avoiding this type of shock hazard is to ensure that the pa-

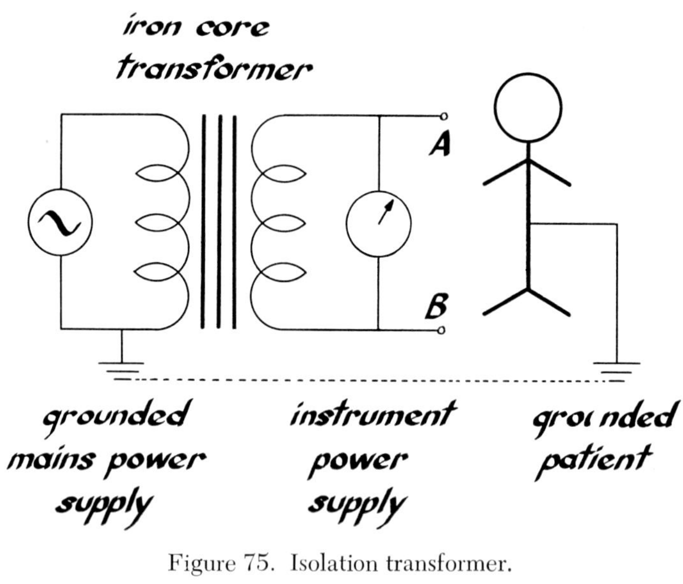

Figure 75. Isolation transformer.

tient is not earthed. However, it is difficult to avoid connection with ground because much of the apparatus surrounding a patient is connected to ground, either directly to the mains power supply ground or indirectly to the true ground itself through the building, plumbing, etc. In some cases the patient is earthed deliberately in order to obtain a reference zero voltage to measure an ECG or EEG. Note that if deliberate grounding is employed, then only one earth connection should be used because the earth of the mains power supply can differ from that of true ground, or even that of other mains power supplies, by several volts.

In an attempt to eliminate this hazard, isolation transformers are used to provide a power supply voltage between two wires (A and B, Figure 75), neither of which is connected to ground. As Figure 75 demonstrates, an earthed patient can contact either A or B (but not both) without becoming part of a circuit with either the generator or the voltage induced in the secondary coil. If, however, the patient touches both A and B, he becomes part of a circuit with the voltage induced in the secondary and experiences a shock.

The isolation transformer appears to be an excellent solution to the shock hazard of the grounded patient, but the description has so far ignored the fact that the primary and secondary coils are coupled by an electric field as well as magnetically. Each coil of the transformer acts as one plate of a capacitor so that alternating currents, albeit small, can flow through the isolating transformer. The currents, called *leakage*, are not large enough to produce a shock hazard normally but can be enough for microshock. Newer types of isolation transformer are designed more rigorously than in the past so as to reduce the leakage current.

ELECTRIC ARC HAZARD

Electric arcs, whether due to static charges accumulated on objects and clothing or to faulty electric circuit connections, constitute a hazard in the presence of explosive mixtures of anaesthetic agents. As explained in Chapter 5 an explosion can be initiated by a relatively small amount of ignition energy, and electric arcs can supply this energy. The arcs occurring in electrical equipment, such as cautery, diathermy, motors, relays, switches and mains power supply sockets, are the responsibility of the electrical engineer for the most part, although the anaesthetist must be aware of the hazard and be alert for faulty equipment. Explosion proof equipment is constructed by sealing it against the anaesthetic mixture, and, together with safety interlock devices (such as mains power sockets which lock the plug in unless the switch is off) and proper maintenance, can almost eliminate the possibility of arcing in electrically operated equipment.

Electric arcs due to static charges are more difficult to eliminate, e.g. static charges build up on nonconducting surfaces (plastics, fabrics, etc.) which preferentially collect positive or negative charges. Providing a low resistance path to ground/earth can eliminate these static charges but also increases the electric shock hazard. Antistatic rubber, identified by a yellow marker, contains carbon black to increase its conductivity and produce a resistance between 50kΩ and 100 MΩ. Terrazzo flooring contains a galvanized steel mesh embedded in it to increase its conductivity to about 2 MΩ (between 2 electrodes 4 in^2, 2 feet apart). These resistance values are a compromise, low enough to conduct static charges but high enough to avoid increasing the electric shock hazard.

Clothing consisting of synthetic fabrics is capable of producing a sizeable static charge; operating room clothing and fabrics are thus made of antistatic cloth like cotton (note that wool is not antistatic). Clothes in contact with the skin have their charges conducted away by the skin surface so that as long as conductive footwear is worn, the charges are led to earth/ground via the floor.

Plastic surfaces which may produce static charges can be sprayed with an antistatic conductive spray to eliminate their arcing hazard in explosive environments, and this principle can be extended to the whole operating room by humidification of the atmosphere. A relative humidity of 70 percent ensures that all surfaces are covered with an invisible film of water which provides a conductive pathway for static charges.

PROBLEM 12

For the circuit shown in Figure 76, $R = 10\text{k}\Omega$ and $C = 1\ \mu\text{F}$, determine the frequency of a sinusoidal input signal V_{in} which results in an output signal $V_{out} = V_{in}/2$. Assume that no current leaves via the output.

Note that this circuit is a simple electrical analogue of a blood pressure canulla with an air bubble (compliance) in it, where V_{in} corresponds to the input blood pressure, and V_{out} corresponds to the pressure detected by a pressure transducer. What do you conclude about the effect of bubbles in cannulas on pressure signal transmission?

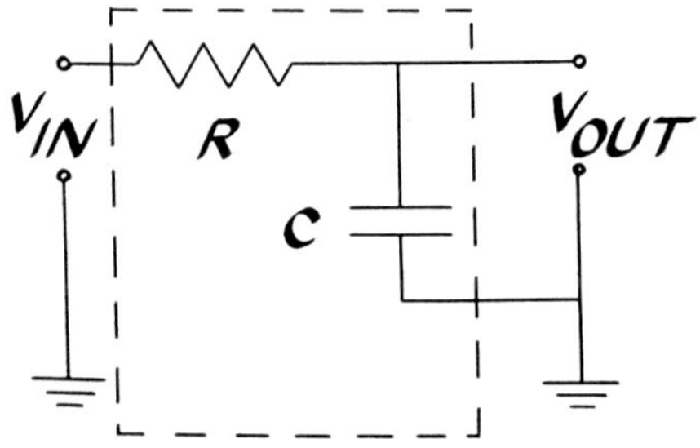

Figure 76. A.C. circuit for Problem 12.

Chapter 13

PATIENT MONITORING

FROM THE VIEWPOINT of instrumentation, a patient becomes a collection of physiological variables to be measured and displayed. Those variables that are not bio-electrical are often transduced into electrical signals because the equipment for the amplification and display of physiological variables is usually electronic. Each stage of transduction, amplification and display has characteristics which affect the correct replication of the measured variable, and so methods of characterizing the signals and their treatment have been developed.

FOURIER'S SERIES

Two sine waves of the same frequency and phase angle add to produce a resultant sine wave, but if either the phase angles or the frequencies differ the resultant wave is not a sine wave, although it does periodically repeat itself. Figure 77 shows a periodic waveform that results from the sum of three sine waves.

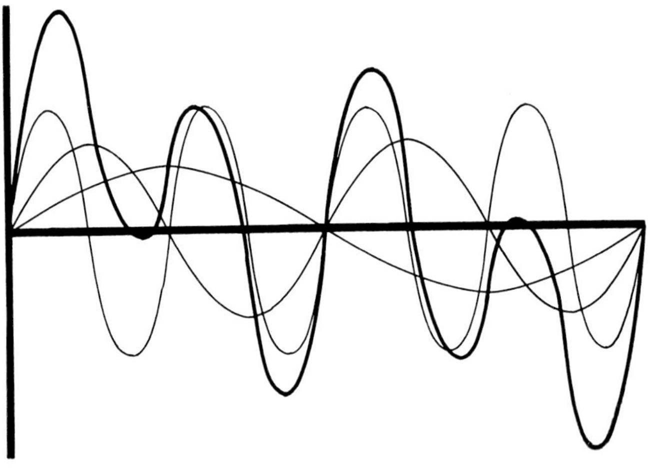

Figure 77. Illustration of Fourier's series.

The phase angles of the three component sine waves are the same but their frequencies differ and are integer multiples of the lowest frequency component sine wave.

This example shows that periodic wave forms can be made by adding sine waves together. Jean Baptiste Joseph Fourier (1763-1830), the French mathematician and physicist, proved that any periodic waveform can be made by adding a series of sine waves together. The amplitudes and phase angles of the sine waves may vary, but the frequencies are integer multiples of the lowest frequency component. The sine wave components are called *harmonics:* first, second, third, etc. The first harmonic and therefore lowest frequency component is also known as the *fundamental.* As well as writing the equation for a periodic waveform as a series of sine wave terms called *Fourier's series;* for example,

$$y(t) = C_0 + C_1 \cdot \sin(2\pi ft + \theta_1) + \cdot C_2 \sin(2\pi 2ft + \theta_2) + C_3 \cdot \sin(2\pi 3ft + \theta_2) + \ldots\ldots$$

where:

$y(t)$ = the periodic waveform,
C_0 = a constant, the D.C. level,
$C_1, C_2, C_3 \ldots$ = the amplitudes of the harmonics,
$\theta_1, \theta_2, \theta_3 \ldots$ = the phase angles of the harmonics,

the series can also be shown graphically as a plot of amplitude versus frequency for each harmonic. The plot is called the *frequency spectrum* of the periodic waveform and contains all of the information in Fourier's series except the phase angles of the harmonics. Figure 78 shows the frequency spectrum for the periodic waveform example of Figure 77.

Although the anaesthetist may encounter some periodic vari-

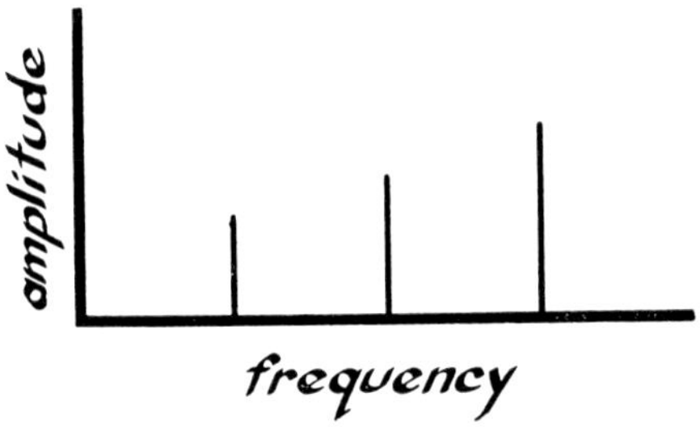

Figure 78. Frequency spectrum.

TABLE XVII

THE FREQUENCY RANGE OF PHYSIOLOGICAL VARIABLES (Hz)

Variable	Range (Hz)
Electrocardiogram	0.1-200
Electroencephalogram	0.5-100
Electromyogram	10-5k
Electro-oculogram	0-120
Electroretinogram	0-10
Galvanic skin potentials	0-0.1
Arterial blood pressure	0-200
Phonocardiography	40-2k
Respiration	0.1-5
Temperature	0-1
Speech sounds	15-20k

ables such as those associated with respiration and circulation, most physiological variables are not periodic waves. Nevertheless, they may still be thought of as a Fourier's series of sine waves, except that the frequency spectrum changes with time. Usually the upper and lower frequency limits of the spectrum are well defined. As a rule of thumb, the number of harmonics and the frequency of the highest harmonic increases with the occurrence of rapid changes in the variable. For example, the ECG waveform has a broader frequency spectrum than that of a respiration waveform.

The concept of Fourier's series enables us to do two things. First, we can describe both electrical signals and physiological variables according to their frequency spectrum. Table XVII lists the range of frequencies for some typical physiological variables. Second, we can represent the characteristics of any signal with a single sine wave whose frequency can vary throughout the frequency range of the signal. Using only a sine wave generator with a variable frequency and amplitude we can test amplifiers and displays. Those that can correctly replicate a sine wave, no matter what its amplitude and frequency within the limits of the frequency spectrum of the signal, will also correctly replicate the signal.

THE BLACK BOX

One of the ways to conceptualize electronic circuits and devices is to view them as black boxes with only the input and out-

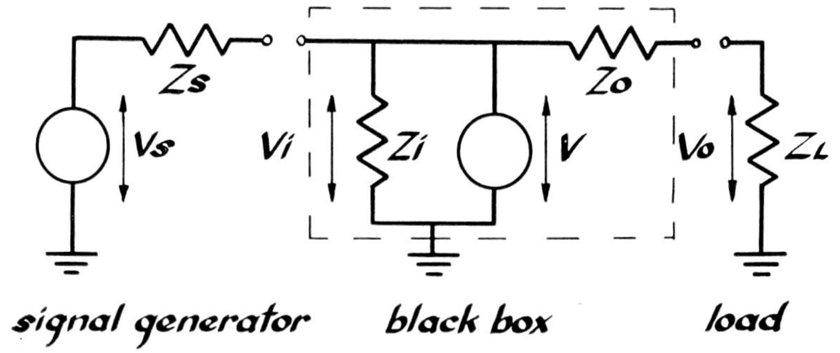

Figure 79. Black box concept.

put terminals accessible. No matter what the black box contains, its contents are envisioned as combinations of ideal elements (pure impedances composed of pure resistance, capacitance and inductance, and ideal generators, constant voltage or constant current).

Figure 79 shows a black box connected to a signal generator and variable load impedance. The signal generator is idealized as a sine wave generator connected to its output terminals through a series, output impedance. Both the signal generator frequency and amplitude can be set by the operator. Using this test circuit we can define the characteristics of the black box and their effect on its performance.

Input Impedance

By measuring the current and voltage at the input terminals of the black box for various signal generator amplitude and frequency settings we can determine the impedance which appears across the input terminals of the black box. It is envisioned as a particular impedance element (pictured in Figure 79 as a resistance) and called the *input impedance.*

From a consideration of Figure 79, it is evident that a small input impedance would cause a large current to be drawn from the signal generator. In this case the power and voltage lost in the signal generator impedance would also be large and little output would reach the black box. Ideally then, the input impedance of the black box should be as large as possible so as to avoid losses in the signal source.

Output Impedance

By setting the input to the black box at some constant value and varying the load impedance we can determine the value of the idealized impedance in series with the black box's generator from measurements of voltage and current made at the output terminals. This impedance is called the *output impedance.* From the previous discussion of input impedance we know that the higher the output impedance the less signal reaches the output terminals, and thus ideally, the output impedance should be as small as possible.

Gain

The black box may either increase the signal passing through it, or decrease it, or leave it unchanged. This effect of the black box is specified by the ratio of output/input in terms of voltage, current or power (voltage and power being more commonly used). If the ratio is greater than one, the black box is called an *amplifier,* and the ratio is referred to as an *amplification factor.* If the ratio is less than one, the black box is called an *attenuator,* and the ratio is referred to as an *attenuation factor.*

The ratio of output/input is often expressed on a logarithmic scale of power in units of bels or decibels (db) and called *gain.* The bel was named in honour of Alexander Graham Bell (1847-1922), the Scottish-Canadian inventor of the telephone, and is defined as the logarithm to the base 10 of the ratio of two powers, that is

$$\text{Gain} = \log_{10}\left(\frac{Pout}{Pin}\right) \text{ bels}$$

$$= 10 \log_{10}\left(\frac{Pout}{Pin}\right) \text{ decibels}$$

where: *Pout* and *Pin* are the *out*put and *in*put powers respectively. From the definition of gain, it can be seen that amplifiers exhibit positive gain while attenuators show negative gain.

The bel scale was originally introduced to specify the subjective loudness of one sound relative to another and is a logarithmic function of the sound power ratio because the subjective output of sensory systems (in this case hearing) is approximately a logarithmic function of the stimulus (recall the Weber-Fechner generalization from Chapter 1). As a scale for gain the decibel has the advantage of compressing a wide variation in the output/input ratio into a manageable scale.

In order to express the output/input ratio of voltage on the gain scale for a black box, it is necessary to assume that the input and output voltages are developed across the same value of resistance. In this case,

$$Pout = \frac{Vout^2}{R},$$

and

$$Pin = \frac{Vin^2}{R};$$

so that,

$$\text{gain} = 10 \log_{10} \left(\frac{Pout}{Pin}\right) = 10 \log_{10} \left(\frac{Vout}{Vin}\right)^2 \text{ db},$$

and

$$\text{gain} = 20 \log_{10} \left(\frac{Vout}{Vin}\right) \text{ db}.$$

Vin and *Vout* are the *in*put and *out*put voltages respectively.

Bandwidth

Ideally the gain of a black box is constant for all frequencies of sine waves, but practically it is approximately constant for only a range of frequencies. Figure 80 shows a plot of gain versus signal generator frequency for a black box which is an amplifier. Note that the frequency scale is logarithmic in order to display a wide range of frequencies.

The range of frequencies over which the gain does not decline from the maximum by more than 3db is called the *bandwidth* of the amplifier. A 3db decline in gain is equivalent to a decline in power output/input ratio by a half, and a decline in voltage ratio by a factor of 0.707.

The importance of bandwidth as a black box specification is that it must exceed the frequency range of any signal passing through it or else the signal will be distorted. For example, suppose that a step change in voltage is applied to the input terminals of a black box. The frequency range of a step change signal extends from zero hertz to very high frequencies, and in order to faithfully replicate the step change signal, the bandwidth of the black box must equal or exceed this frequency range. Note that amplifiers whose bandwidth extends to zero hertz are called *D.C. amplifiers,* and all others are, therefore, *A.C. amplifiers.* As a rule of thumb for D.C. amplifiers, the time taken to complete a step change at the output in response to a step change at the input is the reciprocal of the bandwidth. For example, if a step change from 0 to 2 volts is applied to a D.C. amplifier with a bandwidth of 0 to 20 Hz, and a gain of zero, then the output takes $1/20 = 50$ ms to change from 0 to 2 volts.

So far we have assumed that the black box operates continuously, but some devices act as *samplers,* taking a measurement of the physiological variable or electrical signal for short periods of time only, at a fixed sampling rate (frequency). An example of the action of a sampling unit is shown in Figure 81. The original signal is decoded from the sampled signal by a *demodulator.*

Intuitively we know that if the sampling frequency is too low

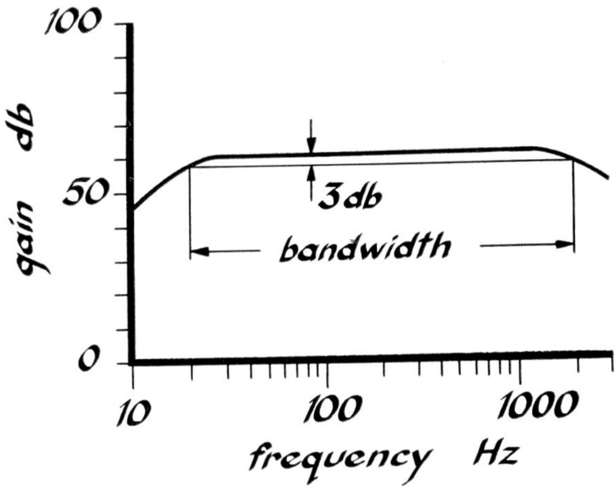

Figure 80. Definition of bandwidth.

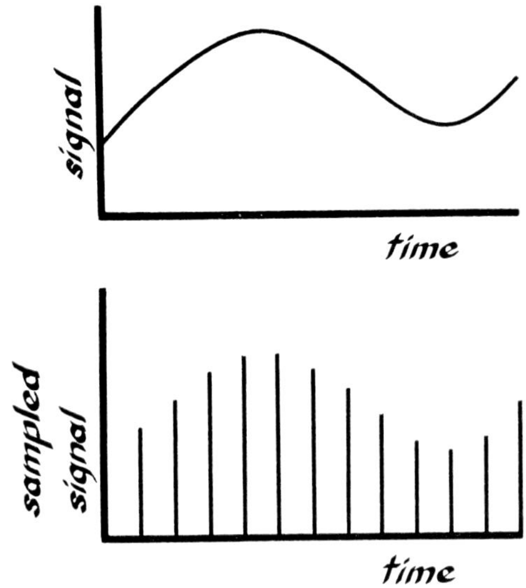

Figure 81. Sampler action.

then some of the rapidly occurring changes in the signal will be missed between samples. Claude Elwood Shannon (1916-), the American mathematician and founder of modern communication theory, determined that the minimum sampling frequency for correct replication of the signal is twice that of the highest signal harmonic.

Signal/Noise Ratio

All electronic devices produce output variations that are unrelated to the input signal and called *noise*. The noise may be generated internally or externally and is usually not large enough to be noticed. However, in critical situations the noise may exceed the signal. The noise performance criterion for any black box is the *signal/noise ratio,* ideally, as large as possible.

Each of the functioning parts of an instrumentation system, transduction, amplification and display, can be evaluated using the black box concept and its performance criteria. Signal sources too can be characterized as analogues of the sine wave generator with its series impedance. The next sections categorize the forms which the black boxes are liable to take as transducers, amplifiers and displays.

TRANSDUCERS

The *transducer* converts physiological variables into electrical signals. Ideally the electrical signal replicates the variable exactly, but in practice the accuracy of reproduction is limited. Although there are a large number of transducer forms, the number of principle operating elements is considerably less. Transducing elements may be divided into two main categories: *active,* generating electrical signals internally, and *passive,* requiring electrical excitation from an external source.

The passive elements are simply resistance, inductance or capacitance elements whose values are altered by the variable to be transduced. Changes in their properties can be detected through their performance in suitable electrical circuits. One of the most commonly used circuits is the *Wheatstone bridge.*

Figure 82a shows the electrical circuit known as the Wheatstone bridge (named after Sir Charles Wheatstone, 1802-1875, the English physicist), as it is usually drawn, and Figure 82b shows a more easily understood identical circuit. Resistance *X* varies with some physiological variable while resistance, *R*, is adjustable. The bridge is used to detect changes in resistance *X* as

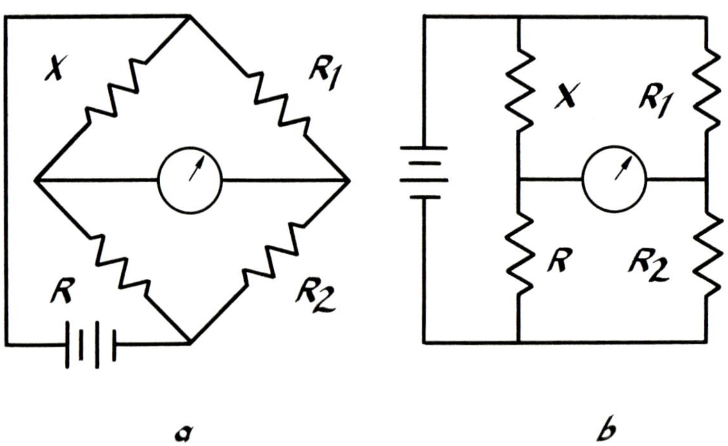

Figure 82. Wheatstone bridge.

follows. With the physiological variable at its zero value and X therefore at its normal resting value, the bridge resistor R is adjusted so that the current through the meter is zero. The bridge is balanced. This condition will only occur when the voltage across R_1 equals the voltage across R_2 and the voltage across X equals the voltage across R; that is, by Ohm's law, when

$$I_1R_1 = I_2R_2 \text{ and } I_1X = I_2R.$$

Dividing the two equations,

$$\frac{I_1X}{I_1R_1} = \frac{I_2R}{I_2R_2},$$

and

$$X = \left(\frac{R_1}{R_2}\right) R.$$

If the ratio R_1/R_2 is known, then the resistance X can be determined from the above equation when R is adjusted to produce zero current in the detector meter. Over small deviations in X, the detector current is linearly related to X, and hence to the physiological variable. For more accurate work over larger variations the bridge may be made self-balancing, and the balancing adjustment is then directly proportional to the change in the physiological variable. Examples of resistance elements used as transducing elements are strain gauges, photoresistors and thermistors.

The above bridge circuit used resistance in a D.C. circuit. A.C. bridges of similar principle are used to detect changes in capacitance and inductance. Instead of a battery, these circuits use sine wave excitation, and instead of balancing just resistance, both resistance and reactance must be adjusted to achieve balance. Many blood pressure transducers are made using a change in inductance detected by an A.C. bridge.

There are a large number of active transducing elements, some of which are listed in Table XVIII with examples of their use.

Transducers form the interface between the variables to be measured and the system of amplification and display. Because they are interface connectors, transducers are the weakest link

TABLE XVIII

TRANSDUCING ELEMENTS

Passive elements:

1. Change of resistance, e.g. stain gauges, photo resistors, thermistors.
2. Change of capacitance, e.g. moving the plates of a capacitor (≡ condenser); as in a condenser microphone.
3. Change of inductance, e.g. moving the core in a coil; as in many pressure transducers.

Active elements:

1. The piezoelectric effect; a crystal generates a voltage across its faces when deformed, e.g. Korotkoff sound microphone.
2. The photoelectric effect; photoelectric materials generate electric charges when illuminated, e.g. the photoelectric cell.
3. The thermoelectric effect; when two metals are joined a temperature dependent voltage is generated across their junction, e.g. thermocouple.
4. The effects of radiation; ions are generated and may be detected, e.g. geiger counter.
5. The electrode potential effect; voltage is generated across the interface of any two material phases (the pH electrode).
6. The Faraday principle of electromagnetic induction (the electromagnetic blood flow meter).

in any measurement system. It is, therefore, important to understand the use and operation of particular transducers according to a set of specifications like those of a black box.

Analogous to an input impedance specification, *Kelvin's first law of instrumentation* states that the measuring instrument must not alter the event being measured. This limitation requires the careful and judicious use of transducers. For example, a pneumotachograph would be useless if its resistance was so high as to cause a noticeable resistance to breathing. If possible the output impedance of a transducer should be low but this performance specification can usually be compensated for by using an amplifier with a very high input impedance.

A transducer should be designed so as to produce an electrical signal that is directly proportional to the input variable within a specified operating range; that is, the graph of output versus input (the calibration curve) should be a straight line. The property is expressed by a performance specification called *linearity*, usually expressed as a percent deviation of the calibration from a straight line. One of the factors affecting linearity

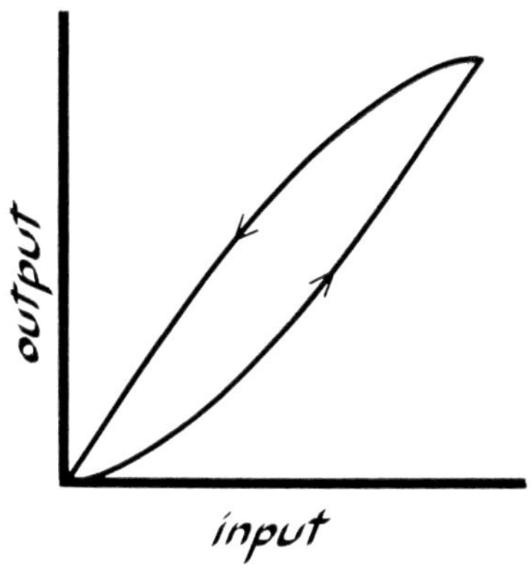

Figure 83. Definition of hysteresis.

is the inability of a transducer to produce an output signal independent of the direction of the change. This behaviour is termed *hysteresis,* and, as Figure 83 illustrates, the calibration graph is a loop.

The frequency response of a transducer must equal or exceed the frequency spectrum of the physiological variable or else the output signal will be a distorted version of the input. If the transducer is a sampler, then the rule of Shannon applies.

AMPLIFIERS

There are no general rules governing the classification of amplifiers, but several terms are normally used to refer to specific types of amplifiers. The most common distinction made between amplifiers is their ability to provide a constant output level in response to a constant input signal. If the amplifier possesses this ability, regardless of how it is achieved, then the amplifier is called a *D.C. amplifier.* If the amplifier does not have this ability, then it is an *A.C. amplifier.*

The next most comprehensive classification refers to the number of input and output terminals. An input or output consisting of two terminals plus a ground/earth terminal, with the signal carried as the difference between the voltages on each terminal with respect to earth/ground, is given the description *differential.* An input or output consisting of one terminal plus an earth/ground terminal, with the signal carried as the voltage with respect to ground/earth, is given the description *single-ended.* The two types of terminal are illustrated in Figure 84, which shows an amplifier with a differential input and a single-ended output.

A major attraction of the differential input is its insensitivity to signals which are simultaneously in phase at both inputs relative to earth/ground. These in-phase signals are usually due to electrical interference such as A.C. hum induced by the mains power lines, and so the differential input configuration can serve to increase the signal/noise ratio of an amplifier. The quality of the in-phase signal rejection is specified by a quantity called the *common mode rejection ratio* which is measured as the magnitude of the in-phase voltage on both terminals relative to ground/

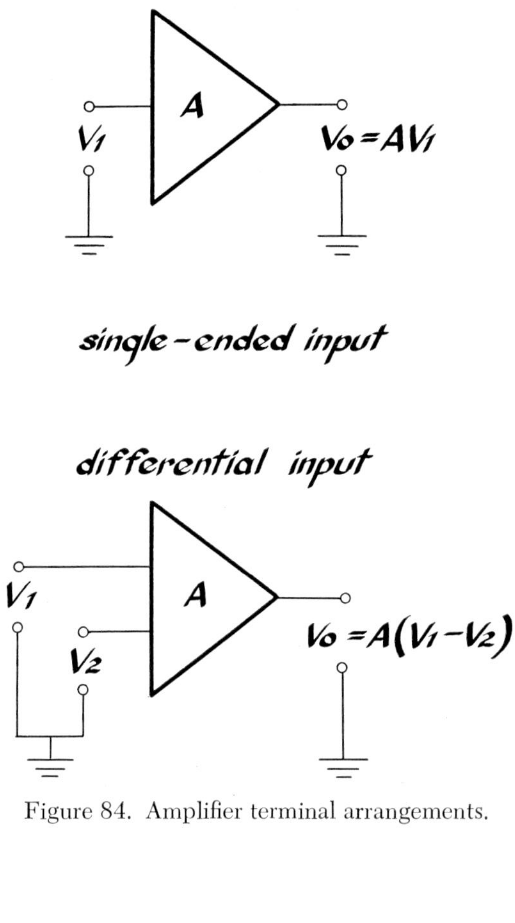

Figure 84. Amplifier terminal arrangements.

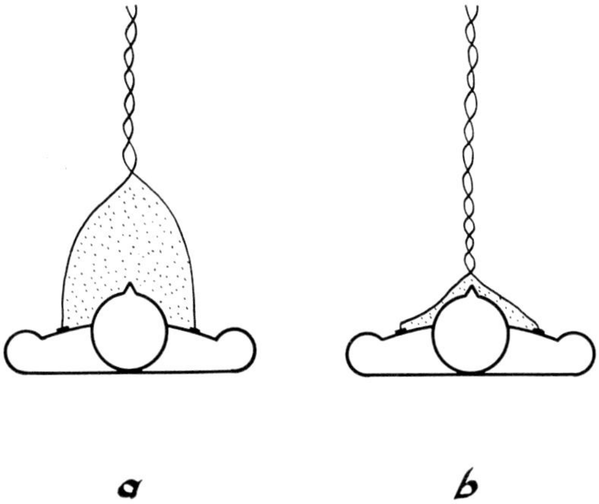

Figure 85. A.C. interference pickup with ECG leads.

earth, divided by the magnitude of the differential voltage required to produce the same amplifier output. Practical values of common mode rejection ratio are of the order of 10^4, which means that signals common to both inputs must be 10^4 times as large as difference signals in order to produce the same output.

One of the most common monitoring problems is the pick-up of A.C. interference, usually by magnetic induction. Figure 85a shows two leads connected to an amplifier for the measurement of an ECG. The leads form a loop which acts like a single turn secondary of a transformer in picking up the A.C. magnetic field from power lines; the induced voltage varies directly as the magnetic field strength and the area of the loop. Therefore, in order to reduce the A.C. interference, the loop formed by the leads should have a minimum area such as is shown in Figure 85b. In addition, the use of a differential input amplifier will reduce the effects of induced A.C. on the output ECG.

The *carrier amplifier* is a specialized type of amplifier operating over a narrow band of frequencies. Figure 86 shows the encoding of a signal by means of *amplitude modulation*. The carrier amplifier is used to amplify the modulated carrier, and so its bandwidth need only be wide enough to pass the encoded waveform. By limiting the bandwidth of the amplifier the signal/noise ratio is improved because noise frequencies outside

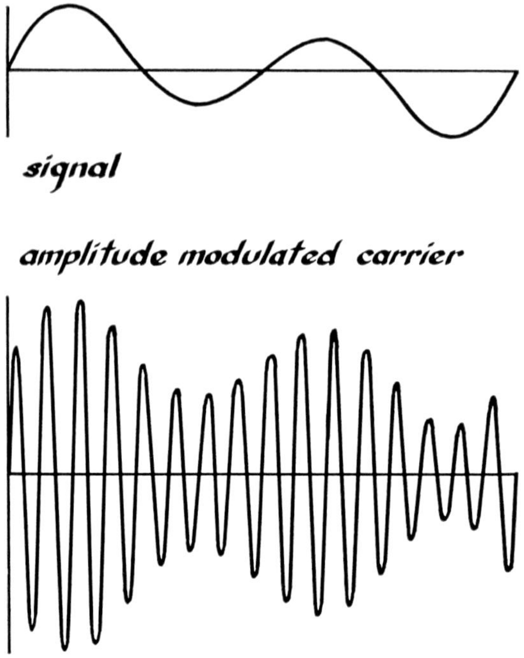

Figure 86. Amplitude modulation.

the *passband* (range of operating frequencies) are not amplified. The carrier amplifier is used extensively with transducers based upon changes in inductance or capacitance, and which therefore require sinusoidal excitation. The amplitude modulation system is very similar to the action of a sampler, and it is not surprising to note that the rule of Shannon applies to the frequency of the carrier with respect to the signal frequency.

The sampling principle itself is used in the construction of stable D.C. amplifiers using the modulation system shown in Figure 87. The D.C. "chopper" amplifier uses a sampler to encode a D.C. signal as an A.C. signal, amplifies the A.C. signal, and then decodes the output to obtain the amplified original D.C. signal. The reason for this rather circuitous method of producing a D.C. amplifier is that by this means a highly stable D.C. amplifier can be produced using a less expensive A.C. amplifier. The name "chopper" refers to the sampler which chops up the signal. A mechanical "chopper" can be detected as an audible buzz. Again, the rule of Shannon applies.

The specifications for the performance of an amplifier are the same as those for the black box. A high input impedance becomes important in such applications as pH meters where the cell voltage to be amplified is produced by only a small movement of charge; thus, any substantial current drain disrupts the cell. The output impedance of an amplifier should be sufficiently low to supply the next stage of instrumentation. The bandwidth of the amplifier must exceed that of the signal to avoid signal distortion. Gain accuracy refers to the agreement of the gain setting with the gain actually obtained. Linearity specifies the variation of the gain with signal amplitude, and the frequency response graph shows the variation in gain at different frequencies.

Two important characteristics which relate to D.C. amplifiers are *offset* and *drift*, which refer to how close the output signal is to zero with no input, and how much this condition changes

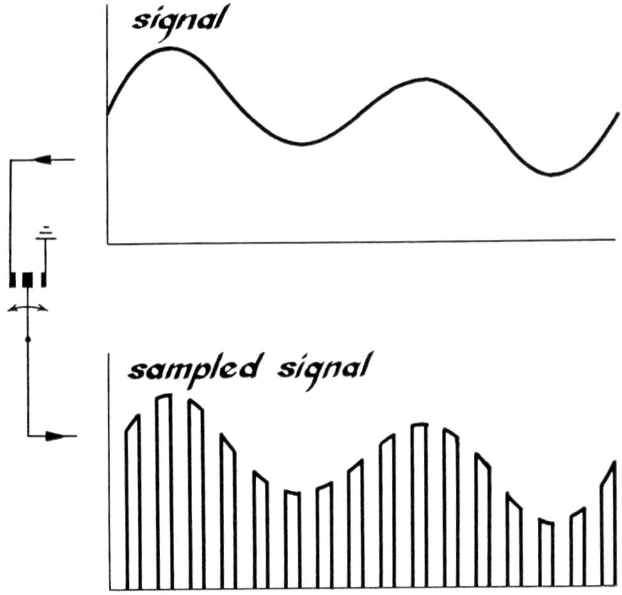

Figure 87. Sampling by chopper.

with time and/or temperature respectively. Offset and drift voltages may be referred to the output or the input. For example, if the offset is 25 μV referred to the input, then the offset for an amplifier with a gain of 10^3 referred to the output would be 25 mV.

RECORDERS

The means of displaying signals visually, and producing permanent records are extremely varied. However, the principles of faithful replication of the signal, analogous to those of transducers and amplifiers, are the same for all types. The following sections classify recorders into types, and review their principles of operation.

Pen Recorders

The pen recorder is essentially a more powerful version of a display meter, the pen arm replacing the pointer. The pen motor consists of a coil with an iron core suspended in the field of two large permanent magnets. The signal current passes through the coil, and the resultant magnetic field interacts with the field of the permanent magnet to turn the pen by an amount proportional to the signal. The motor may also be constructed with a moving permanent magnet and fixed coils. The pen traces an arc whose distance from a fixed zero line is proportional to the signal. Depending upon the construction of the pen motor, the bandwidth may vary from 0 to 2 Hz to 0 to 100 Hz, the upper frequency being limited by the inertia of the pen arm and coil.

Several methods of writing are used for pen recorders; the cheapest is untreated paper and ink pens. Ink feeds may be by capillary syphoning or by pressurization; all types require care to avoid clogging. Other writing systems include pressure sensitive paper and paper sensitive to an electrically charged pen. The hot stylus method uses specially treated paper covered with white cellulose. The heat burns off the cellulose and exposes a black underlayer to create the trace.

The heated stylus system is used so as to produce a rectilinear trace rather than an arc like a conventional pen. Figure 88a shows how the elongated heated stylus contacts the paper only at a knife edge and so writes rectilinearly. The other method of

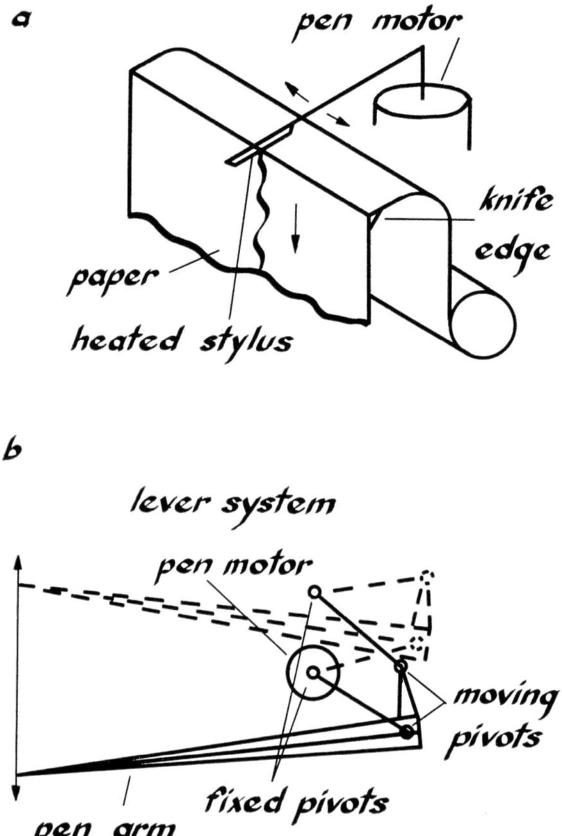

Figure 88. Production of a rectilinear trace.

producing a rectilinear trace is to use a lever system as shown in Figure 88b. The levers operate to extend the length of the pen arm so that the arc traced approximates a straight line.

Galvanometer Recorders

The galvanometer is essentially a moving coil device like a pen motor, but the pen arm is replaced by a light beam so that the coil need only turn a tiny mirror. The reduction in the size and inertia of the moving coil yields a much higher bandwidth. Figure 89 shows the schema of operation.

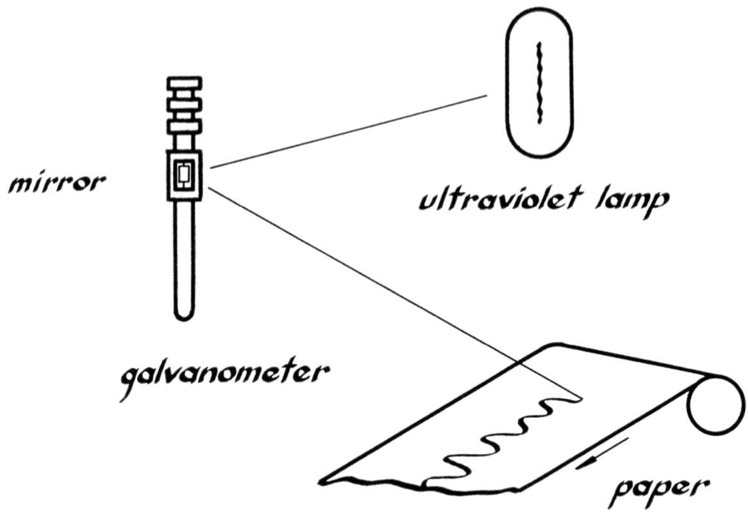

Figure 89. Operation of a galvanometer recorder.

Originally this type of recorder wrote with a beam of visible light on photographic film. However, the requirements of film developing limited its popularity, and alternate methods were sought. One type of modern galvanometer recorder writes with a beam of ultraviolet light generated by a mercury vapour lamp on paper which develops its trace upon exposure to light. Continuous exposure overdevelops the trace, so the record must be stored in the dark, or wet processed, or sprayed with a yellow stabilizing lacquer. Ultraviolet (UV) recorders have bandwidths as high as 0 to 10 kHz.

Another type of galvanometer recorder uses an ink jet instead of a light beam. The galvanometer coil turns a tiny nozzle instead of a mirror. A pressure system jets the ink on to ordinary paper. The jet feed system requires careful adjustment so as to avoid excessive inking at low paper speeds. Bandwidths up to 0 to 700 Hz can be obtained with ink jet recorders.

Potentiometric Recorders

The potentiometric recorder is in principle a self-balancing precision potentiometer. Figure 90 shows how it works. A *po-*

tentiometer is formed by a high resistance wire connected across the width of the paper record and a moving contact (wiper) which picks off the voltage at its point of contact. For example, with the voltage across the wire as 10 volts, the wiper would pick off a voltage somewhere between zero and ten volts depending upon its position along the wire. The wiper carries the pen and is motor driven so as to take up any position along the wire. The motor is energized by a signal which is the difference between the input voltage and the wiper voltage. Such a control system is called a negative feedback servomechanism. The pen moves to a position where the wiper voltage equals the input voltage and thereby traces the input signal on paper. The servomechanism may be simple, as illustrated here, or it may be complex and exploit control system technology to the full.

The potentiometric recorder may also be used to control pen motion along what is normally the time axis controlled by the paper transport mechanism. In this case, the pen moves in both X and Y directions, and the recorder is called an XY recorder. Graphs of one signal versus another signal instead of time may be made using an XY recorder, e.g. pressure versus volume to determine the work of breathing. The potentiometric recorder is not a high frequency machine, however, due to its high inertia, and so bandwidths of only a few hertz can be obtained.

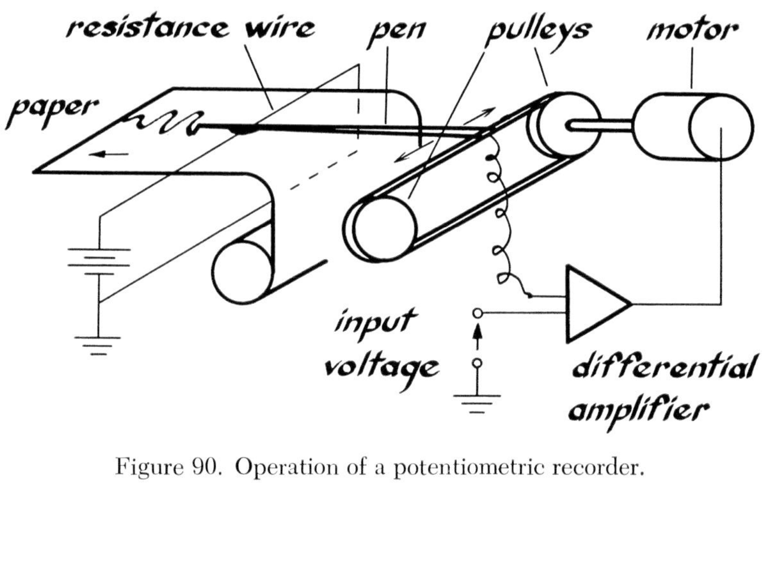

Figure 90. Operation of a potentiometric recorder.

The Cathode Ray Oscilloscope

Although the oscilloscope in both its conventional small screen size and large screen display size is mostly used for display only, the trace can be photographed; it can thus be considered as a recorder too. The basis of the scope or CRO is shown in Figure 91.

Electrons are produced at the *cathode* (negatively charged electrode) by a process of *thermionic emission* (electrons are emitted more easily from a surface coated with special materials and heated). The electrons are attracted by a positively charged electrode (the *anode*) and are accelerated towards it by the electrostatic force of several thousand volts. Other electrodes specially shaped and charged to various voltages create specific electrostatic fields which focus the electron stream into a narrow beam. The whole set of cathode, anode and focussing electrodes is called an *electron gun*. The electron gun shoots a narrow beam of electrons (the *cathode ray*) through a hole in the anode towards a phosphor-coated screen where upon impingment the energy is converted to light, and we see a bright dot on the screen. The electron gun and screen are contained entirely within an

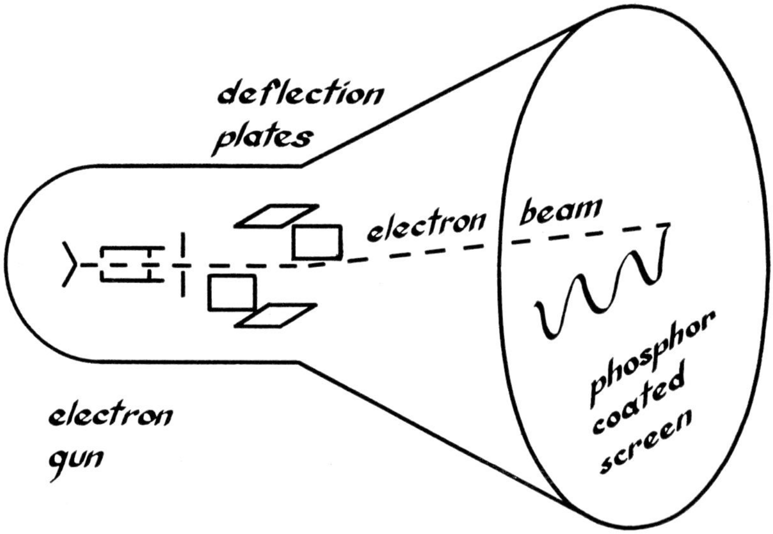

Figure 91. Operation of an oscilloscope.

evacuated glass envelope (the cathode ray tube) so that the electron beam does not collide with gas molecules.

In addition to an electron gun, the cathode ray tube contains horizontal and vertical *deflection plates.* These are sets of electrodes which electrostatically deflect the beam in the horizontal and vertical directions in response to external signal voltages. Usually the horizontal deflection plates are operated with a saw toothed waveform so as to sweep the beam from left to right at a constant rate (thereby forming a time axis) then quickly return the beam right to left to start another sweep. The beam is blanked (turned off) during the return, and only the left to right sweep is seen. The signal to be viewed is applied to the vertical deflection plates so that the screen shows a continuous plot of the signal versus time. The oscilloscope has the widest bandwidth of any recording and display device, from 0 Hz to gigahertz frequencies.

PROBLEM 13

Briefly list the type of amplifier, its characteristics and the type of recorder that you would choose for recording an E.M.G. State the reasons for your choice.

Chapter 14

GAS ANALYSIS

THE MEASUREMENT of constituent concentrations of specific gases in gas mixtures and of blood gas tensions may be accomplished by a wide variety of methods such as:

1. the chemical absorption of sample constituents by the serial application of reagents noting:
   (a) changes in the sample volume at constant temperature and pressure (Haldane, Scholander);
   (b) changes in the sample pressure at constant volume and temperature (Van Slyke)
2. differences in density of gases (Waller's chloroform balance)
3. differences in thermal conductivity of gases (katharometers)
4. differences in refractive index of light for gases (the Rayleigh refractometer)
5. differences in the rate of passage of a gas through a micro-orifice, Graham's law (effusiometers)
6. differences in the velocity of sound in gases
7. differences in the viscosity of gases
8. differences in the magnetic susceptibility, Pauling principle (paramagnetic oxygen analyzer)
9. differences in the wavelength of electromagnetic radiation (light), emitted under electrical excitation (the nitrogen meter)
10. differences in the absorption of electromagnetic radiation (the infrared CO_2 analyser, the ultraviolet halothane analyzer)
11. gas chromatographic separation of mixture components
12. mass spectrometry
13. electrode systems (CO_2 and O_2 electrodes)

Some of these methods may be made to provide continuous

measurements while others are restricted to samples; most employ transducing elements. The methods of gas analysis most frequently used in instruments employed by anaesthetists are optical methods for gases and electrode systems for blood gases.

OPTICAL GAS ANALYSERS

Electromagnetic Radiation—Light

Electromagnetic radiation consists of mutually perpendicular waves of magnetic and electrical field energy. The frequency spectrum of electromagnetic energy includes light, radio waves, X rays and gamma rays. The waves are characterized by their frequency or wavelength. For example, radio waves have wavelengths measured in metres, but light is of higher frequency and wavelengths correspondingly shorter so that the unit of light wavelength is the Angstrom unit ($1Å = 10^{-10}m$). The product of frequency and wavelength equals the velocity of the wave, and for all electromagnetic radiation the velocity in vacuum is constant at approximately 300 Mm/s (the speed of light).

The electrons associated with the atoms of any substance are positioned in a series of specific energy bands or shells. Light, i.e. electromagnetic energy, is capable of causing electrons to jump to a higher energy shell, providing that the energy of the light is exactly the required amount. Since the energy of an electromagnetic wave depends directly upon its frequency, this means that for a particular substance, light of a specific wavelength is required to cause electrons to jump to a higher energy shell. This wavelength of light is absorbed. Use is made of such absorption specificity in optical gas analysers. Note that the reverse of absorption may occur. Electrons, excited to a higher energy state by some means, emit light energy (of a specific wavelength) when they drop back to their normal energy state. If all the electrons drop back together a *laser* effect (light amplification by stimulated emission of radiation) is produced.

Infrared Gas Analysers

With the exception of oxygen and nitrogen, most of the gases and vapours of respiratory and anaesthetic interest have characteristic absorption bands in the infrared region of the spectrum. (Carbon monoxide, carbon dioxide, nitrous oxide, ether, halothane, chloroform and cyclopropane). The construction of an infrared gas analyser usually follows the scheme shown in Figure 92.

Two equal strength beams of infrared light, one passing through the analysis cell, the other unimpeded, fall one on to each half of a detector cell. The detector cell is filled with the gas to be analysed so that it can only absorb those infrared wavelengths which can be absorbed by the sample in the analysis cell. In this way the analyser is made highly selective. The detector cell, a condenser microphone assembly, is a glass cell separated into two halves by a thin flexible metal diaphragm. The diaphragm is the moveable plate of a capacitor and its displacement is detected as a change in capacitance. Because the detector cell is heated less on the analysis side, the difference in pressure pushes the diaphragm to one side. The beams of infrared light are interrupted (chopped), at about 25 Hz or more, by a motor turning a segmented disc, so that the diaphragm alternately flexes and relaxes creating an A.C. signal. The signal is amplified and displayed. Note that Shannon's sampling theorem applies, so that the bandwidth of the CO_2 changes which may be mon-

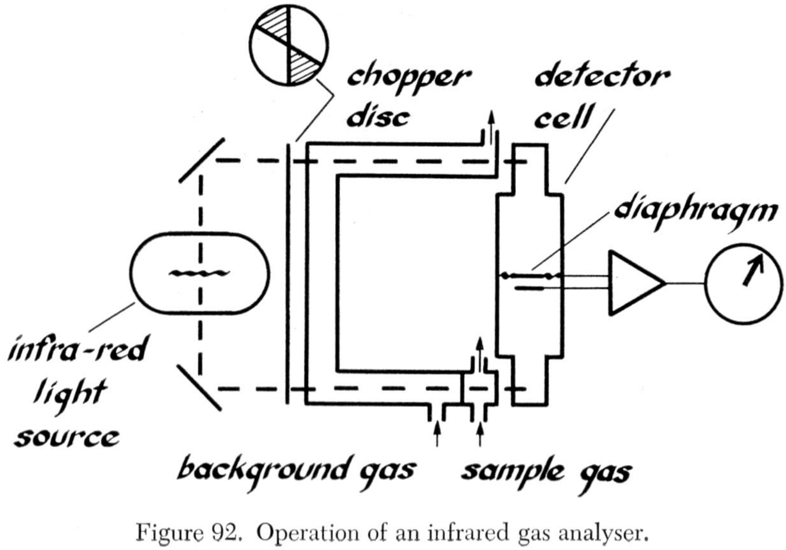

Figure 92. Operation of an infrared gas analyser.

itored is from 0 to 12.5 Hz with a 25 Hz chopper. The reciprocal of the bandwidth (in this case, 1/12.5 Hz = 80 ms), is the time that the analyser output takes to change in response to a step change in CO_2.

The Ultraviolet Halothane Analyser

Halothane exhibits considerable absorption in the ultraviolet region of the spectrum between 2000 and 2700 Å and, since ultraviolet light is more energetic than infrared light, a simpler transducer may be used, in a scheme similar to that of the infrared analyser. Ultraviolet light is generated with a small mercury vapour discharge lamp and falls on to a pair of photocells, one of which has an analysis cell in front of it. The analysis cell is fitted with quartz windows since ordinary glass will not pass ultraviolet. The difference between the two photocell voltages, caused by halothane vapour in the analysis cell attenuating the light to one cell by absorption, is detected and amplified electronically.

The Oximeter

The oximeter, which measures the percent saturation of blood with oxygen, also makes use of optical absorption. A schema of its construction is shown in Figure 93. In the red region of the spectrum at 6500 Å there is a large difference in the optical absorption between haemoglobin and oxyhaemoglobin. If blood is lighted by an incandescent lamp and either the light intensity transmitted or reflected is measured with a cadmium sulphide photoconductive cell, masked by an optical filter which selects the correct wavelength, then the photocell output will vary with the oxygen saturation of the blood. This measurement must be compared to a reference to eliminate haematocrit and source intensity variations. Such a reference is obtainable because in the near infrared region of the spectrum at 8000 Å an isobestic point exists where the optical absorption of haemoglobin and oxyhaemoglobin are equal. A suitable optical filter masking another cadmium sulphide photoconductive cell provides the reference which varies with haemotocrit and source intensity. The difference between the two photocells varies only with oxygen saturation.

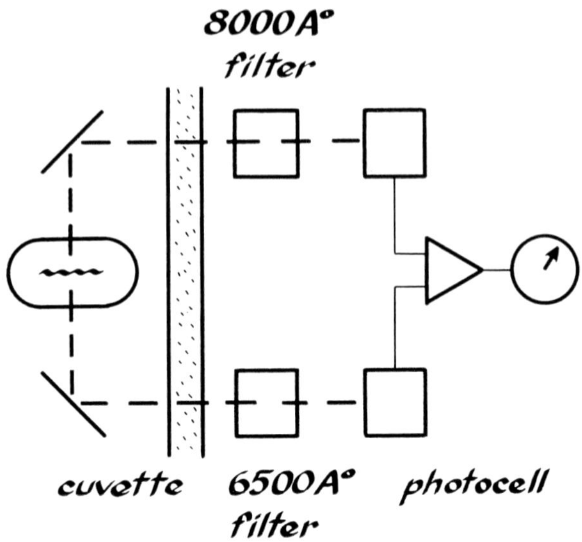

Figure 93. Operation of an oximeter.

The Nitrogen Meter

The nitrogen meter is based upon the fact that nitrogen molecules can be excited in a low pressure electric discharge to emit visible light in the purple region. A small fraction of the sample is passed through a 1500 volt discharge tube by a vacuum pump. Optical filters select the appropriate wavelengths and the light intensity is then measured with a photocell and amplifier. A rotating disc chops the light beam to produce an A.C. signal.

The Paramagnetic Oxygen Analyser

Oxygen may be measured by utilizing the fact that it is *paramagnetic* (a weak form of magnetism compared to *ferromagnetism*), and attracted to a magnetic field. All other gases except nitric oxide are *diamagnetic* (repelled by a magnetic field).

The analyser, diagrammed in Figure 94, operates as follows. A glass dumbbell filled with nitrogen is suspended in a nonuniform magnetic field within the analysis cell containing the oxygen concentration to be measured. Since oxygen molecules are paramagnetic they accumulate between the magnet poles push-

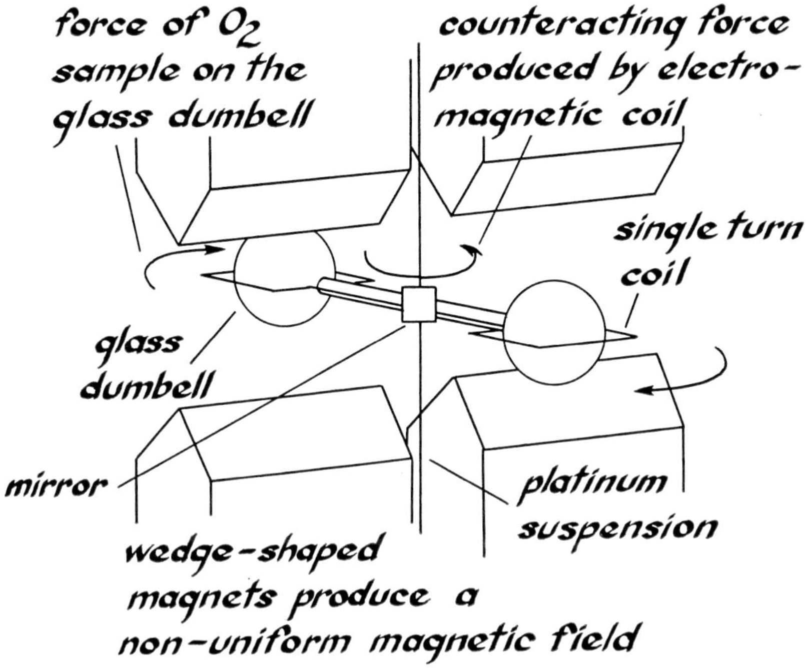

Figure 94. Operation of a paramagnetic oxygen analyser.

ing aside the dumbbell which is not paramagnetic. A tiny mirror, attached to the suspension reflects a beam of light on to a scale. If the dumbbell is returned to its initial position by a counteracting magnetic field produced by passing current through a coil around the dumbbell, then the current is proportional to the oxygen concentration. Note that water vapour dilutes the effect and the gas must be carefully dried. This instrument, unlike the previous analysers, does not respond quickly enough to measure breath by breath changes (in its commercial form).

The Mass Spectrometer

This instrument is perhaps the most sophisticated of all the gas analysers. It is capable of measuring single breath changes simultaneously in a number of gases (usually 4, oxygen, carbon dioxide, nitrogen and one other tracer such as argon). Figure 95

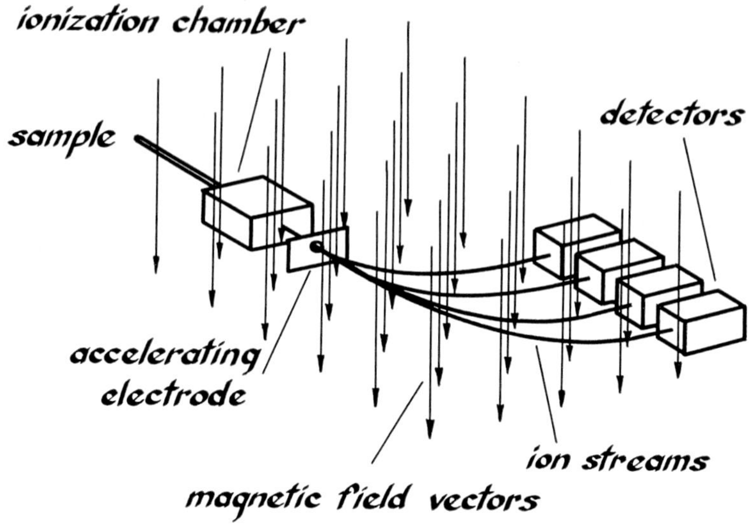

Figure 95. Operation of a mass spectrometer.

shows how it works. The sample stream of gas is ionized in a low pressure electric discharge and the ions are accelerated in an electric field by an amount directly proportional to their charge and inversely proportional to their mass. A magnetic field at right angles to the accelerating electric field (direction of ion stream), deflects the ions by an amount dependent upon their charge and speed. Detectors, placed to intersect the ions characteristic of each gas, measure the electric charge which accumulates and which is proportional to the concentration of each gas in the sample.

ELECTRODE SYSTEMS

Electrode Potential

In order to understand the measurement of the concentration of ions in solution it is necessary to examine the concept of the electrode potential which is produced at the interface between any two material phases. Consider the interface between a metal and an electrolyte. Two processes are in equilibrium: the passage of ions from the metal into solution and the combination of metallic ions in solution with electrons in the metal to form atoms of the metal. A charge gradient results, which takes a form called the electrical double layer, a complex organization of electrical charges immediately adjacent to the electrode. In its simplest form the double layer has been pictured as two parallel sheets of positive and negative charges (Figure 96).

Practically, the electrode-electrolyte interface resembles a voltage source and a large capacitance in parallel with a resistance. The values of these components are not constant and are nonlinearly dependent upon such factors as temperature, electrolyte concentration, type of metal, etc. The voltage developed at an electrode-electrolyte interface is called the *half-cell potential,* so that the total voltage between a pair of electrodes is the sum of the two half-cells formed at each interface. It is impossible to measure the half-cell potential alone since two electrodes are required to measure a voltage, so an arbitrary standard half-cell has been chosen, and half-cell potentials are measured with respect to it. The standard is the hydrogen electrode. Typical half-cell potentials measured in this way are listed in Table XIX. Note that all electrodes for bio-electric events (EEG, ECG, etc.) generate electrode potentials when in contact with biological materials.

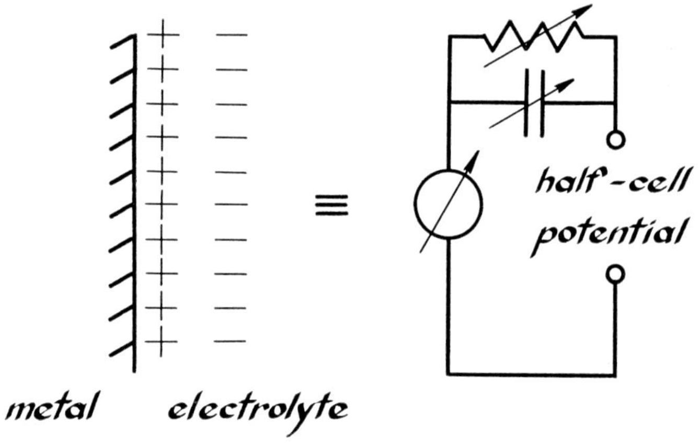

Figure 96. Electrode potential.

TABLE XIX
HALF CELL POTENTIALS*

Element	*Electrode Reaction*	*Potential*† *(Volts)*
Lithium	$Li \rightleftarrows Li^+ + e^-$	−3.05
Potassium	$K \rightleftarrows K^+ + e^-$	−2.93
Calcium	$Ca \rightleftarrows Ca^{++} + 2e^-$	−2.87
Sodium	$Na \rightleftarrows Na^+ + e^-$	−2.71
Magnesium	$Mg \rightleftarrows Mg^{++} + 2e^-$	−2.37
Aluminium	$Al \rightleftarrows Al^{+++} + 3e^-$	−1.66
Manganese	$Mn \rightleftarrows Mg^{++} + 2e^-$	−1.18
Zinc	$Zn \rightleftarrows Zn^{++} + 2e^-$	−0.76
Iron	$Fe \rightleftarrows Fe^{++} + 2e^-$	−0.44
Nickel	$Ni \rightleftarrows Ni^{++} + 2e^-$	−0.25
Tin	$Sn \rightleftarrows Sn^{++} + 2e^-$	−0.14
Lead	$Pb \rightleftarrows Pb^{++} + 2e^-$	−0.13
Hydrogen gas	$H_2 \rightleftarrows 2H^+ + 2e^-$	0
Copper	$Cu \rightleftarrows Cu^{++} + 2e^-$	+0.34
Silver	$Ag \rightleftarrows Ag^+ + e^-$	+0.80
Mercury	$Hg \rightleftarrows Hg^{++} + 2e^-$	+0.85
Platinum	$Pt \rightleftarrows Pt^{++} + 2e^-$	+1.20
Gold	$Au \rightleftarrows Au^{+++} + 3e^-$	+1.50

* L. H. Cragg and R. P. Graham: *An Introduction to the Principles of Chemistry.* Clarke, Irwin and Company, Limited, Toronto, Canada.

† Standard electrode potentials measured at 25°C relative to the hydrogen electrode potential as zero. Ionic concentrations are 1 mol/litre.

The Nernst Equation

A liquid-liquid interface may be formed by placing a semi-permeable membrane, which allows reversible transfer of one particular ion, between two liquids. After equilibrium has been established, the potential created is proportional to the logarithm of the ratio of the concentrations of the ion to which the membrane is selectively permeable. For a membrane which is ideally selective, the potential developed is given by the equation stated by Walter Nernst (1864-1941), the German physical chemist.

$$E = \frac{-RT}{nF} \cdot \ln \frac{C_1}{C_2},$$

where:

E = the potential in volts,
R = the universal gas constant,
n = the valence of the ion,

T = absolute temperature,
F = coulombs of charge transferred,

and

C_1 and C_2 = concentration of the selected ion on each side of the membrane.

In the practical case, departure from ideal thermodynamic behaviour is expressed in terms of the ionic activity rather than ionic concentration.

$$a = C \cdot A,$$

where:

a = the activity of a specific ion,
C = the ionic concentration,

and

A = the activity coefficient.

The Nernst equation becomes:

$$E = \frac{-RT}{nF} \cdot \ln \frac{a_1}{a_2} .$$

Activity coefficients must be known if the ion concentration is to be determined in terms of the electrical potential developed. Note that if a membrane exhibits a selective permeability to a particular type of ion then it provides the means of making a transducer for that particular ion.

Reference Electrodes

Since the measurement of ionic concentrations depends upon the determination of the liquid-liquid interface potential and this can only be measured by using metal electrodes, thereby creating half-cells, then the reference voltage of the half-cells must be stable and accurate. The standard or reference electrode previously mentioned was the hydrogen electrode.

Hydrogen is a gas, but electrical connection to it may be made as follows (Figure 97). A platinum wire or plate is electrolytically coated with finely divided platinum (platinum black) to increase its surface area. The platinized wire or plate readily absorbs hydrogen and is itself a good conductor. When this electrode is immersed partially in a solution containing hydrogen ions and hydrogen is blown past the uncovered portion of the electrode, a difference in potential, depending on the tendency of the gas to go into solution and on the concentration of hydrogen ions in solution, will develop.

In theory, the hydrogen electrode could be used to measure the pH of solutions, but is has obvious disadvantages as a practical reference electrode and as a pH electrode. Therefore, half-cells of high stability and convenience are normally used as electrodes to measure liquid-liquid interface potentials. The most practical are the calomel and the silver-silver chloride electrodes.

In the calomel electrode the potential is developed across a junction of pure mercury and a solution of potassium chloride which is saturated with mercurous chloride (calomel), as shown in Figure 98. The potential depends upon the concentration of potassium chloride used.

The measurement of the potential of other interfaces using the calomel half-cell as a reference often gives rise to a liquid-liquid interface. Such liquid-liquid potentials may be minimized by the use of a salt bridge, consisting of a saturated solution of potassium chloride held in agar gel in a glass tube. The salt bridge connects the calomel potassium chloride solution to the liquid phase of the half cell to be measured. Potassium and

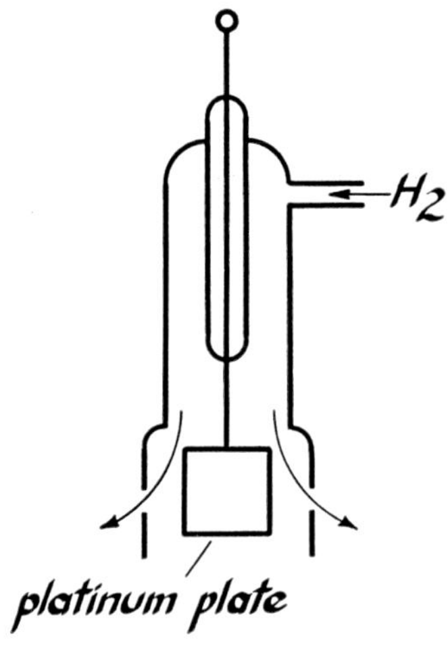

Figure 97. Hydrogen electrode.

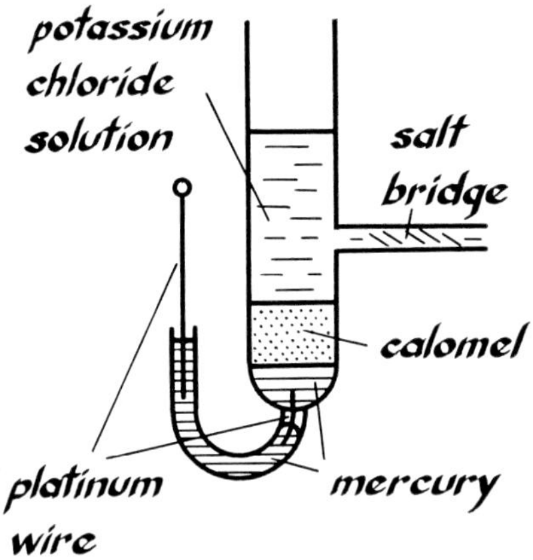

Figure 98. Calomel electrode.

chloride ions have approximately the same mobilities, and hence minimize the formation of concentration gradients and resulting electrical potentials. A substitute, if KCl cannot be used due to the presence of ions, e.g. silver which may produce undesirable chemical reactions, is ammonium nitrate. The calomel electrode, besides its ease of construction and use, has the advantage of long term stability. Note that because ionic mobilities are temperature dependent the half-cell voltage is also temperature dependent (0.0059 volts/°C for a +0.28 volt cell).

The silver-silver chloride electrode is made by electroplating silver with chloride ions which combine to produce a silver chloride coating (chloriding). The electrode has the advantage of being easy to prepare, reproducible and small. Like the calomel electrode the half-cell potential depends upon the concentration of the potassium chloride solution, which it contacts, and the temperature.

The pH Electrode

The discovery of a glass membrane, which permits the passage of hydrogen ions only (in the form of H_3O^+), made possible a pH electrode. The thin glass membrane may be in the form of a spherical bulb or a capillary tube. Inside the glass membrane a buffered solution of HCl contacts an Ag-AgCl electrode. Outside is the solution of unknown pH. Connection from this unknown solution to an electrode is made via a salt bridge and a calomel half-cell. The voltage between the mercury and silver is about 60 millivolts per unit of pH at 30°C. The interfaces of the pH meter shown in Figure 99 are:

Ag · AgCl/Chloride buffer/glass/solution of unknown pH//Saturated KCl//Hg_2Cl_2 · Hg

where:

/ = solid-liquid interface and // = liquid-liquid interface.

The Nernst equation applied to the pH electrode system is:

$$V \propto RT \cdot \ln \frac{[H^+]b}{[H^+]s},$$

where:

V = voltage between mercury and silver,
R = universal gas constant,
T = temperature in degrees absolute,
$[H^+]b$ = buffer hydrogen ion concentration,

and

$[H^+]s$ = sample hydrogen ion concentration.

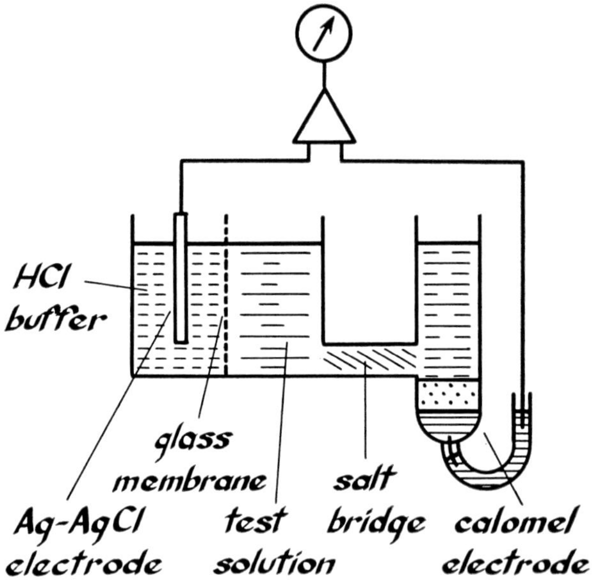

Figure 99. pH meter.

Note that the temperature and the buffer hydrogen ion concentration must be kept constant in order to keep the voltage dependent upon the sample pH only.

Some limitations of the glass electrode are as follows: The pH range over which accurate response is obtained may be restricted unless special glasses are used. The measurement of the potential must be made with a high input impedance device, since the potential is developed by the movement of relatively few ions across a glass membrane. The glass electrode shows a loss in sensitivity and a decreased speed of response after a period of service (especially when used in solutions containing proteins), which may be restored by etching the surface to remove the inactive outer layer.

The Pco_2 Electrode

In 1957 Stow described the Pco_2 electrode. It was a standard pH electrode covered with a membrane permeable to CO_2. Between the membrane and the glass was a thin film of water which equilibrated with the Pco_2 of the test solution outside the membrane. After equilibration the pH of the film of water was measured and the Pco_2 determined from the linear relationship

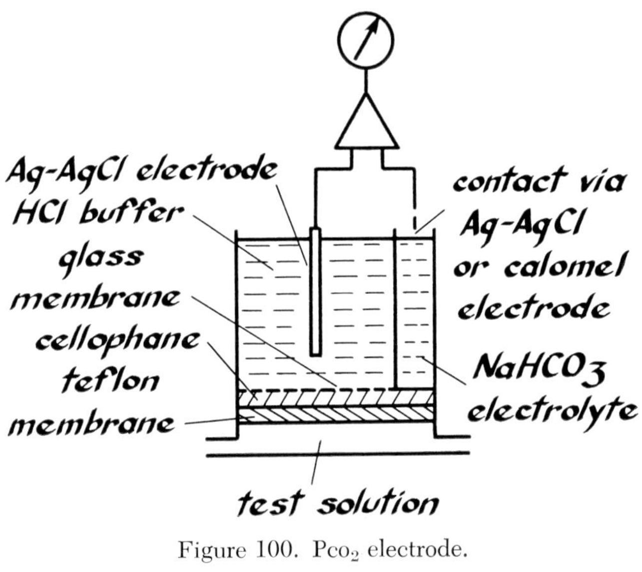

Figure 100. Pco_2 electrode.

between log Pco_2 and pH described by the Henderson-Hasselbalch equation.

Several modifications of the original electrode have been introduced which have increased the sensitivity, stability and response time. Bicarbonate ion added to the water film increased the sensitivity. Teflon membrane was substituted for the original rubber membrane. A cellophane spacer membrane was introduced to hold the water film on the glass and then later replaced by fibres of glass wool. A typical CO_2 electrode is shown in Figure 100.

Measurement of blood Pco_2 may be made with a pH electrode alone, using the Astrup method. Three pH measurements are taken, the sample directly, and two similar samples equilibrated with two different standard gas mixtures of known Pco_2, e.g. 60 and 30 mm Hg. A nomogram of log Pco_2 vs pH is employed to yield the sample Pco_2, standard bicarbonate, base excess, and buffer base.

The Po_2 Electrode

The oxygen electrode is a glass coated platinum wire whose tip cross-sectional area is exposed to the solution in which the Po_2 is to be measured. Connection to the solution is made via a salt bridge and an Ag · Ag Cl reference half-cell. If a voltage of about 0.2 volts is applied between the silver and the platinum wires so as to make the platinum negative (cathode), then oxygen from the solution reaching the surface of the platinum is reduced electrolytically, i.e. O_2 accepts electrons to provide charge movement. Electric current is thus in the circuit. When the platinum is made more negative (−0.6 to −0.9 volts) the rate of electrolytic reduction, and thus the amount of current which can flow, is limited by the rate at which O_2 can diffuse to the surface. Since the rate of diffusion is proportional to the Po_2 of the solution (Fick), then the current in the circuit is proportional to the Po_2 in the body of the solution.

Oxygen electrodes suffer from two main problems: aging and the diffusion field. *Aging* is the slow reduction in current over a period of time even though the Po_2 of the solution is kept constant. It is associated with material attaching itself to the electrode surface. To combat aging the current may be reversed

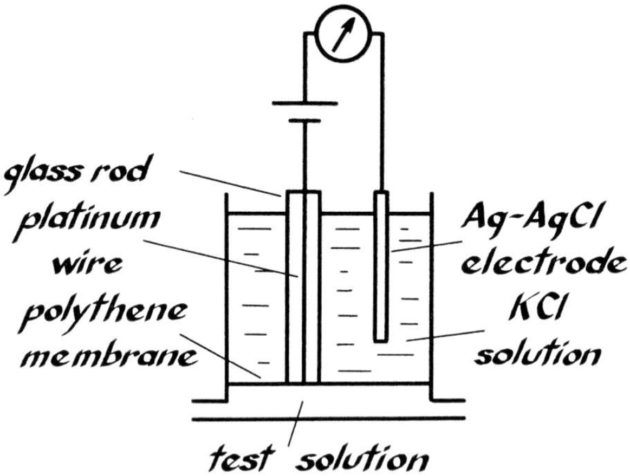

Figure 101. Po_2 electrode.

periodically, and the electrode may be covered with a protective film such as polythene. The second problem associated with the oxygen electrode is the fact that the electrode operates by reducing O_2 and so gives rise to a *diffusion field* about the electrode. The Po_2 in the vicinity of the electrode may be less than that which would exist if the electrode were not present. This source of error may be minimized by constantly moving the solution past the electrode.

The Clark type of oxygen electrode, schematically pictured in Figure 101, utilizes a self-contained Ag-Ag Cl reference half-cell (electrode), which contacts the saturated KCl solution surrounding the platinum electrode. The platinum electrode and a thin layer of KCl solution are separated from the solution to be measured by a polythene membrane. The stability of this form of oxygen electrode depends upon the diffusion distance between the platinum surface and the membrane, and therefore it must be kept taut.

The Westinghouse Oxygen Monitor

This oxygen monitor for gas analysis uses two solid///solid half cells: Platinum///zirconium oxide///platinum, as shown in Figure 102.

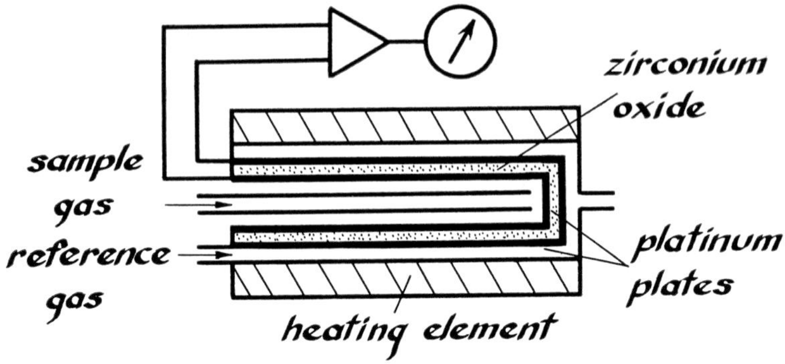

Figure 102. Westinghouse oxygen monitor.

The cells are operated at 850°C so as to obtain a measureable cell voltage. The partial pressure of oxygen at each platinum/zirconium oxide interface determines the half-cell voltage since the interchange of charges for a half-cell is:

$$O_2 + 4e \rightleftarrows 2O^=$$

Gaseous oxygen plus electrons from the platinum flow from the platinum to the ZrO_2 to form two oxygen ions in one direction; oxygen ions from the oxide meanwhile flow to the platinum, releasing electrons and gaseous oxygen in the opposite direction. The Nernst equation for the cell is

$$V = 55 \log_{10} (Pr/Ps),$$

V = the voltage developed by the cell,
Pr = the Po_2 of the reference gas,
Ps = the Po_2 of the sample gas.

Note that ordinary rusting occurs because and by the oxidation process described here.

BIBLIOGRAPHY

1. Adriani, J.: *The Chemistry and Physics of Anesthesia,* 2nd ed. Springfield, Thomas, 1970.
2. Crul, F. J. and Payne, J. P. (Eds.): *Patient Monitoring.* Amsterdam, Exerpta Medica, 1970.
3. Hill, D. W.: *Principles of Electronics in Medical Research,* 2nd ed. London, Butterworths, 1973.
4. Hill, D. W.: *Physics Applied to Anaesthesia,* 2nd ed. London, Butterworths, 1972.
5. Hill, D. W.: *Electronic Measurement Techniques in Anaesthesia and Surgery.* London, Butterworths, 1970.
6. Macintosh, R.; Mushin, W. W., and Epstein, H. G.: *Physics for the Anaesthetist,* 3rd ed. Oxford, Blackwell, 1970.
7. Mushin, W. W.; Rendell-Baker, L.; Thompson, P. W., and Mapleson, W. W.: *Automatic Ventilation of the Lungs,* 2nd ed. Oxford, Blackwell, 1969.
8. Nunn, J. F.: *Applied Respiratory Physiology.* London, Butterworths, 1969.
9. Scurr, C. F. and Feldman, S. A.: *Scientific Foundations of Anaesthesia.* London, Heinemann, 1970.
10. Sykes, M. K. and Vickers, M. D.: *Principles of Measurement for Anaesthetists.* Oxford, Blackwell, 1970.

Appendix I

SOLUTIONS TO PROBLEMS

1(a). Figure 103 shows the relationship

$$y = \frac{1}{x}$$

plotted on rectagular coordinates from the following table of values:

y	x
± 5	$\pm 1/5$
± 4	$\pm 1/4$
± 3	$\pm 1/3$

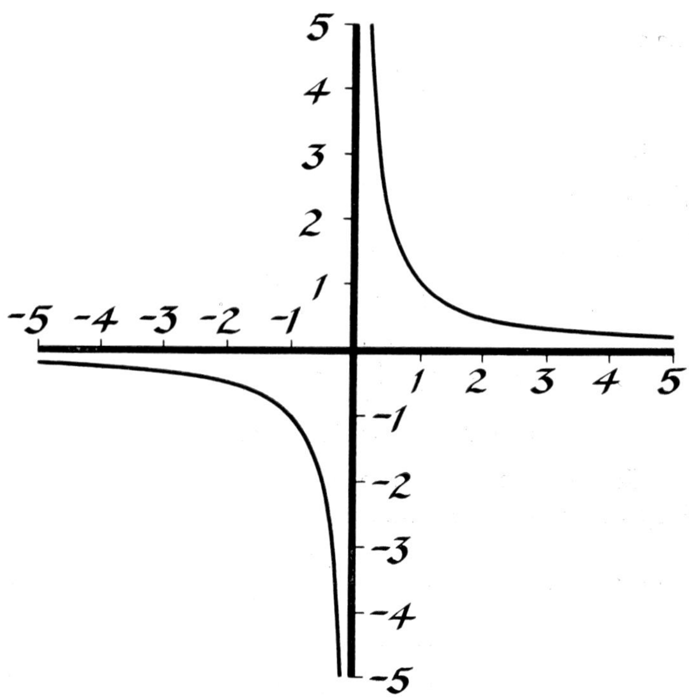

Figure 103. Plot of the equation $y = 1/x$.

± 2	$\pm 1/2$
± 1	± 1
$\pm 1/2$	± 2
$\pm 1/3$	± 3
$\pm 1/4$	± 4
$\pm 1/5$	± 5

1(b). The stroke volume of the sine wave ventilator is $2 \times 250 = 500$ ml. The frequency in Hz is

$$f = \omega / 2\pi = 0.6\pi / 2\pi = 0.3 \text{ Hz.}$$

Since 1/3 of a cycle occurs in a second, one cycle or breath takes three seconds. Breathing rate is $60/3 = 20$ breaths/minute.

2(a). The equation,

$$y = 3x^3,$$

is of the form, $y = Kx^n$, and therefore the differentiation formula,

$$\frac{dy}{dx} = Knx^{n-1},$$

may be applied:

$$\frac{dy}{dx} = 3\,(3x^2),$$

for $x = 2, \frac{dy}{dx} = 3 \times 3 \times 2 \times 2 = 36.$

The slope of the curve, $y = 3x^3$ at $x = 2$ is 36 units/unit.

2(b). The integration formula is

$$\int y \cdot dx = \frac{Kx^{n+1}}{n+1}.$$

Therefore, $${}_2\!\int^4 3x^3 = \left[\frac{3x^4}{4}\right]_2^4 = \frac{3 \times 4^4}{4} - \frac{3 \times 2^4}{4}$$

$$= 192 - 12 = 180 \text{ square units.}$$

3(a). In a constant pressure generator the volume rises exponentially with a time constant RC to a final volume, CP.

$$\text{Time constant} = RC = 10\ \frac{\text{cm } H_2O \cdot \text{sec}}{\text{litre}} \times 50\ \frac{\text{ml}}{\text{cm } H_2O}$$

$$= 500 \text{ ml} \cdot \text{sec/litre}$$

$$= 500 \text{ ml} \cdot \text{sec/1000 ml}$$

$$= .5 \text{ sec}$$

$$\text{Final volume} = CP = 10 \text{ cm } H_2O \times 50 \frac{\text{ml}}{\text{cm } H_2O}$$
$$= 500 \text{ ml}$$

Pressure applied for 0.5 sec, i.e. one time constant, so 63.2 percent of the final volume is attained according to Figure 20:

$$\text{i.e. } 500 \text{ ml} \times 0.632 = 316 \text{ ml delivered}$$

Pressure applied for 2 sec, i.e. four time constants, so 98.2 percent of the final volume is attained:

$$\text{i.e. } 500 \text{ ml} \times .982 = 491 \text{ ml delivered.}$$

If the resistance doubles, the time constant doubles to one sec.

Pressure applied for .5 sec, i.e. ½ time constant, so 39 percent of the final volume is attained:

$$\text{i.e. } 500 \text{ ml } (1 - e^{-0.5/1}) = 500 \ (1 - 0.607)$$
$$500 \text{ ml} \times .39 = 195 \text{ ml delivered.}$$

Pressure applied for two seconds, i.e. two time constants, so 86.5 percent of the final volume is attained:

$$\text{i.e. } 500 \text{ ml} \times .865 = 433 \text{ ml delivered}$$

3(b). In a constant flow generator the volume rises linearly with a slope, F, of 250 ml/sec.

Volume delivered in 0.5 sec is

$$0.5 \text{ sec} \times 250 \frac{\text{ml}}{\text{sec}} = 125 \text{ ml}$$

Volume delivered in 2 sec is

$$2 \text{ sec} \times 250 \frac{\text{ml}}{\text{sec}} = 500 \text{ ml}$$

If the resistance doubles, the volumes remain the same.

4. Convert to S.I. units:

$$V_T = 500 \text{ cm}^3$$

$$100 \text{ cm} = 1 \text{ m so } 10^6 \text{ cm}^3 = 1 \text{ m}^3$$

$$V_T = 500 \text{ cm}^3 \times \frac{1 \text{ m}^3}{10^6 \text{ cm}^3} = 5 \times 10^{-4} \text{ m}^3$$

and

$$C = 100 \frac{\text{cm}^3}{\text{cm H}_2\text{O}} \times \frac{\text{lm}^3}{10^6 \text{ cm}^3}$$

$$= 10^{-4} \text{ m}^3/\text{cm H}_2\text{O}$$

The pressure of 1 cm H_2O column is = height × density × G.

$$\text{density of H}_2\text{O} = 1 \frac{\text{g}}{\text{cm}^3} \times \frac{1 \text{ kg}}{10^3 \text{ g}} \times 10^6 \frac{\text{cm}^3}{1 \text{ m}^3} = 10^3 \text{ kg/m}^3$$

$$\text{acceleration due to gravity, } G = 9.81 \text{ m/sec}^2$$

$$\text{column height} = 1 \text{ cm} = 10^{-2}\text{m.}$$

Therefore, pressure of 1 cm H_2O is equal to

$$10^{-2}\text{m} \times 10^3 \frac{\text{kg}}{\text{m}^3} \times 9.81 \frac{\text{m}}{\text{s}^2}$$

$$= 98.1 \frac{\text{kg} \cdot \text{m}}{\text{s}^2 \cdot \text{m}^2} = 98.1 \text{ N/m}^2 = 98.1 \text{ Pa}$$

$$C = 10^{-4} \frac{\text{m}^3}{\text{cm H}_2\text{O}} \times \frac{1 \text{ cm H}_2\text{O}}{98.1 \text{ N/m}^2} = \frac{10^{-4} \quad \text{m}^3}{98.1 \text{ N/m}^2}$$

$$= 1.02 \times 10^{-6} \frac{\text{m}^3}{\text{Pa}}$$

For 1 breath,

$$\text{P.E.} = V^2/2C = \frac{25 \times 10^{-8} \text{ m}^6}{2.04 \times 10^{-6} \text{ m}^3/\text{Pa}}$$

$$= 0.123 \text{ N} \cdot \text{m} = 0.123 \text{ Joules}$$

For 1 hour,

$$\text{P.E.} = 0.123 \frac{\text{Joules}}{\text{breath}} \times 15 \frac{\text{breaths}}{\text{min.}} \times 60 \frac{\text{min.}}{\text{hr.}}$$

$$= 110 \text{ Joules/hr.} = 110 \frac{\text{Joules}}{\text{hr.}} \times \frac{1 \text{ hr.}}{60 \text{ min.}} \times \frac{1 \text{ min.}}{60 \text{ s}}$$

$$= 0.03 \text{ watts average.}$$

5(a). temperature change of blood is 35°C − 10°C = 25°C 1 g of blood raised through 25°C requires 0.87 cal./g °C × 25°C = 21.75 cal./g. Blood flow is

$$100 \text{ ml/min.} \times 1 \text{ min./60 s} = 1.67 \text{ ml/s}$$

or

$$1.67 \text{ ml/s} \times 1.06 \text{ g/ml} = 1.77 \text{ g/s.}$$

So the heat flow is

$$1.77 \text{ g/s} \times 21.75 \text{ cal./g} = 38.5 \text{ cal./s}$$

or

$$\begin{aligned} & 38.5 \text{ cal./s} \times 4.184 \text{ J/cal.} \\ & = 161 \text{ J/s} \\ & = 161 \text{ W} \end{aligned}$$

Power rating of water heater is, therefore

$$161 \text{ W}$$

Heat flow could be increased by 1) increasing the water temperature; 2) increasing the area of the blood-water interface.

5(b). $\dot{V}_E$ = 6 l/min. = 6000 ml/min. In the Boyle's apparatus the loss of H_2O vapour is 6% of 6 l/min.

i.e. 360 ml/min.

$$\text{or } 360 \frac{\text{ml}}{\text{min.}} \times \frac{1 \text{ g}}{1400 \text{ ml}} = .257 \text{ g/min.}$$

The heat loss is

$$.257 \frac{\text{g}}{\text{min.}} \times 539 \frac{\text{cal.}}{\text{g}} = 138.5 \text{ cal./min.}$$

In the circle system the loss of H_2O vapour is 6% − 2% = 4%

Heat loss is proportionately less

$$138.5 \frac{\text{cal.}}{\text{min.}} \times \frac{4\%}{6\%} = 92.3 \text{ cal./min.}$$

6(a). Let V_E = the expired gas volume, litres
T_A = the ambient temperature, K
P_B = the barometric pressure, mm Hg
P_{H_2O} = the partial pressure of water vapour, mm Hg

The ideal gas law:

$$\frac{P_1V_1}{T_1} = \frac{P_2V_2}{T_2}.$$

$$P_1 = P_B - P_{H_2O}, \; P_2 = 760 \text{ mm Hg}$$

$$V_1 = V_E \quad V_2 = V_{STPD}$$

$$T_1 = T_A \quad T_2 = 273 \text{ K}$$

$$\frac{(P_B - P_{H_2O})V_E}{T_A} = \frac{760\ V_{STPD}}{273}$$

$$V_{STPD} = V_E(P_B - P_{H_2O})\frac{273}{760\ T_A}$$

6(b). Adiabatic compression: $P_1V_1^\gamma = P_2V_2^\gamma$
$V_1 = 60\text{ l} \quad V_2 = 59.5\text{ l}$
$P_1 = 1033 \text{ cm } H_2O \quad P_2 = ?$

$$P_2 = \frac{P_1\dot{V}_1^\gamma}{V_2^\gamma}$$

$P_2 = 1033\ (60/59.5)^{1.41}$

$\log 60 = \log(6.0 \times 10) = 1 + 0.7782 =$	1.7782
$\log 59.5 = \log(5.95 \times 10) = 1 + 0.7745 =$	1.7745
$\log(60/59.5) = \log 60 - \log 59.5 =$	0.0037
	× 1.41
$\log(60/59.5)^{1.41} = 1.41 \times \log(60/59.5) =$	0.0052
$\log 1033 = \log(1.033 \times 10^3) = 3 + 0.0140 =$	3.0140
$\log P_2 = \log(1033\ (60/59.5)^{1.41} =$	3.0192

antilog: $P_2 = 1045 \text{ cm } H_2O$

Compliance is

$$500/(1045 - 1033) = 41.7 \text{ ml/cm } H_2O.$$

Isothermal compression:

$$P_1V_1 = P_2V_2$$

$$P_2 = \frac{P_1V_1}{V_2}$$

$$P_2 = \frac{1033 \times 60}{59.5} = 1042 \text{ cm } H_2O$$

Compliance is

$$\frac{500}{(1042 - 1033)} = 55.5 \text{ ml/cm } H_2O$$

7(a). *METHOD 1*

6 l/min. total flow; 1% is halothane vapour flow, i.e. 60 ml/min. at 20°C, 760 mm Hg pressure. At 20°C, 760 mm Hg, 1 mole of halothane vapour occupies 24.0 litres. The molar flow of halothane is

$$.06 \frac{\text{litres vapour}}{\text{min.}} \times \frac{1 \text{ mol}}{24.0 \text{ litres vapour}}$$

$$= 2.5 \times 10^{-3} \text{ moles/min.}$$

But the gram molecular weight of halothane is 197 g/mol, therefore the mass flow of halothane is

$$2.5 \times 10^{-3} \frac{\text{mol}}{\text{min.}} \times 197 \frac{\text{g}}{\text{mol}} = 0.492 \text{ g/min.}$$

Since the liquid density of halothane is 1.86 g/ml the flow of halothane liquid is

$$0.492 \frac{\text{g}}{\text{min.}} \times \frac{1 \text{ ml}}{1.86 \text{ g}} = 0.265 \text{ ml/min.}$$

METHOD 2

A 1% halothane vapour concentration means that the partial pressure of halothane vapour is 7.6 mm Hg. The minute volume flow is 6 l.

$$PV = nRT$$

R = 62 mm Hg · l/mol K
T = 293 K
n = ?
V = 6 l
P = 7.6 mm Hg

$$n = \frac{7.6 \text{ mm Hg} \times 6 \text{ l} \times \text{mol} \times \text{K}}{62 \text{ mm Hg} \times \text{l} \times 293 \text{ K}}$$

$$n = 2.5 \times 10^{-3} \text{ moles}$$

The molar flow of halothane is, therefore,

$$2.5 \times 10^{-3} \text{ mol/min.}$$

Continue as for method 1.

7(b). In the vaporizing chamber halothane vapour is at saturation concentration, i.e. at 20°C, a partial pressure of 241 mm Hg. The minute volume at a partial pressure of 7.6 mm Hg is 6 litres.

$$P_1V_1 = P_2V_2$$

$$7.6 \text{ mm Hg} \times 6 \text{ litres} = 241 \text{ mm Hg} \times V_2$$

$$V_2 = \frac{7.6 \times 6}{241} = 0.189 \text{ litres}$$

The flow of halothane vapour from the vaporizing chamber is 189 ml/min.

7(c). For every gram of liquid halothane vaporized at 20°C, 37 calories must be supplied. Heat flow is, therefore,

$$37 \frac{\text{cal.}}{\text{g}} \times 0.492 \frac{\text{g}}{\text{min.}}$$

$$= 18.2 \text{ cal./min.}$$

Since 4.184 J = 1 calorie, the heat flow is

$$18.2 \frac{\text{cal.}}{\text{min.}} \times 4.184 \frac{\text{J}}{\text{cal.}}$$

$$= 76 \text{ J/min.}$$

$$= 76 \frac{\text{J}}{\text{min.}} \times \frac{\text{min.}}{60 \text{ s}}$$

$$= 1.2 \text{ J/s or watts.}$$

The power of a heater to supply the required heat is 1.2 W.

7(d). Since the flow of liquid halothane is 0.265 ml/min., in one hour

$$0.265 \times 60 = 15.9 \text{ ml is vaporized.}$$

8(a). A 1% concentration of halothane in alveolar air means a partial pressure of 7.6 mm Hg. The concentration of halothane in alveolar air in moles per litre may be found using the ideal gas law.

$$PV = nRT$$

$$\frac{n}{V} = \frac{P}{RT} = \frac{7.6 \text{ mm Hg} \cdot \text{mol. K}}{62 \text{ mm Hg} \cdot \text{l} \cdot 310 \text{ K}}$$

$$\frac{n}{V} = 0.395 \text{ m mol/l}$$

$$\lambda_{37°\text{C}} \text{ for blood} = 2.34 \text{ from Table XV}$$

$$\text{i.e. } \frac{(n/V) \text{ blood}}{(n/V) \text{ gas}} = 2.34$$

Therefore, assuming equilibrium between alveolar air and blood,

$$(n/V) \text{ blood} = 2.34 \times 0.395 = 0.925 \text{ m mol/l}$$

$$\lambda_{37°\text{C}} \text{ for olive oil} = 224 \text{ from Table XV}$$

$$\text{i.e. } \frac{(n/V) \text{ olive oil}}{(n/V) \text{ gas}} = 224$$

Therefore, assuming that brain tissue has the same solubility coefficient as olive oil, and assuming that brain tissue is in equilibrium with alveolar air via the bloodstream,

$$\begin{aligned}(n/V) \text{ brain tissue} &= 224 \times 0.395 \\ &= 88.5 \text{ m mol/l}\end{aligned}$$

8(b). A 0.9 g/100 ml NaCl solution is a $0.9/58 = 1.55 \times 10^{-2}$ mol/100 ml solution. If the NaCl was 100 percent ionized the solution would be isosmotic with a glucose solution of $2 \times 1.55 \times 10^{-2} = 3.1 \times 10^{-2}$ mol/100 ml. The NaCl is, however, only about 90 percent ionized, and so the solution is isosmotic with a glucose solution of $3.1 \times 10^{-2} \times .9 = 2.79 \times 10^{-2}$ mol/100 ml, which is a solution of $180 \times 2.79 \times 10^{-2} = 5$ g/100 ml.

8(c). Case 1 isosmotic, isotonic
Case 2 isosmotic, hypotonic
Case 3 isosmotic, hypertonic
Case 4 not isosmotic, isotonic

8(d). Graham's law applies to the effusion of gases through porous membranes.

$$\begin{aligned}\text{diffusion speed} &\propto 1/\sqrt{\text{molecular weight}} \\ O_2 \text{ diffusion speed} &\propto 1/\sqrt{32} \propto 0.177 \\ N_2O \text{ diffusion speed} &\propto 1/\sqrt{44} \propto 0.151\end{aligned}$$

The N_2O diffusion speed is, therefore,

$$\frac{(0.177 - 0.151) \times 100}{0.177}$$

$$= 14.7\% \text{ slower than that of } O_2.$$

9. The cross-sectional area of the tube at the 2 cm diameter section is

$$A_1 = \frac{\pi D^2}{4} = \frac{3.14 \times 0.02 \text{ m} \times 0.02 \text{ m}}{4} = 3.14 \times 10^{-4} \text{ m}^2$$

at the 4 cm diameter section is

$$A_2 = \frac{\pi D^2}{4} = \frac{3.14 \times 0.04 \text{ m} \times 0.04 \text{ m}}{4} = 12.56 \times 10^{-4} \text{ m}^2$$

The average velocity of the water in the 2 cm diameter section is, according to the continuity equation,

$$\bar{v}_1 = \frac{F}{A_1} = \frac{1 \times 10^{-3} \text{ kl/s}}{3.14 \times 10^{-4} \text{ m}^2}$$

$$= 3.18 \text{ m/s}$$

at the 4 cm diameter section:

$$\bar{v}_2 = \frac{F}{A_1} = \frac{1 \times 10^{-3} \text{ m}^3/\text{s}}{12.56 \times 10^{-4} \text{ m}^2}$$

$$= 0.795 \text{ m/s}$$

From the frictionless form of the general energy equation:

$$\frac{P_1}{\rho} + \frac{\bar{v}_1^2}{2} = \frac{P_2}{\rho} + \frac{\bar{v}_2^2}{2}$$

$$P_2 = \rho\left(\frac{P_1}{\rho} + \frac{\bar{v}_1^2}{2} - \frac{\bar{v}_2^2}{2}\right)$$

ρ water from Table XVI is 10^3 kg/m^3

$$P_1 = 5 \text{ mm Hg} \times 133 \frac{\text{Pa}}{\text{mm Hg}} = 665 \text{ Pa}$$

$$\bar{v}_1^2 = 3.18 \times 3.18 = 10.1 \text{ m}^2/\text{s}^2$$

$$\bar{v}_2^2 = 0.795 \times 0.795 = 0.632 \text{ m}^2/\text{s}^2$$

Substituting

$$P_2 = 10^3 \left(\frac{665}{10^3} + \frac{10.1}{2} - \frac{0.632}{2}\right)$$

$$= 10^3 \ (0.665 + 5.05 - 0.316)$$

$$= 10^3 \times 5.399 = 5399 \text{ Pa}$$

or

$$\frac{5399}{133} = 40.6 \text{ mm Hg}$$

The pressure in the 4 cm diameter section is 40.6 mm Hg. This device is called a *diffuser,* and it converts the energy of flow velocity into pressure. In actual practice, frictional effects in the fluid, and the occurrence of eddys dissipating energy will reduce the efficiency of this energy conversion considerably.

10(a). The critical flow for air in tubes is

$$F_c(\text{l/min.}) = 14 \times \text{diameter in cm.}$$

One inch diameter tubing is 2.54 cm, therefore the critical flow for air is

$$14 \times 2.54 = 35.6 \text{ l/min.}$$

Since the peak flow is 25 l/min., the flow is laminar, and the Hagen-Poiseuille law applies.

$$\text{Pressure drop} = 128\ \mu LF/\pi D^4$$

$$\mu = 1.83 \times 10^{-5} \text{ Pa} \cdot \text{s from Table XVI}$$

$$L = 2 \text{ m}$$

$$F = \frac{25 \times 10^{-3} \text{ kl} \cdot \text{min.}}{\text{min.} \times 60 \text{ s}} = 4.17 \times 10^{-4} \text{ m}^3/\text{s}$$

$$D = 2.54 \times 10^{-2} \text{ m};\ D^4 = 4.16 \times 10^{-7} \text{ m}^4$$

The pressure drop in two metres of one inch diameter tubing is

$$\frac{128 \times 1.83 \times 10^{-5} \times 2 \times 4.17 \times 10^{-4}}{3.14 \times 4.16 \times 10^{-7}} = 1.49 \text{ Pa},$$

or

$$1.49 \times 10.2 \times 10^{-3} = 0.0151 \text{ cm } H_2O,$$

in other words a negligible pressure loss.

10(b). Assuming laminar flow:

$$R = \frac{P_1 - P_2}{F} = \frac{128\ \mu L}{\pi D^4}$$

$$F = \frac{P_1 - P_2}{R}$$

Flow may be doubled by doubling $P_1 - P_2$; that is, the height of the bag, or by halving R. The resistance may be halved by increasing the needle bore D. Increase in $D^4 = 2$. Increase in $D = 2^{1/4} = 1.189$ times.

11(a). If resistors R_1 and R_2 are connected in parallel to a battery of voltage E, then the voltage across both resistors will be E. According to Ohm's law, the currents through the resistors will be

$$I_1 = \frac{E}{R_1},$$

and

$$I_2 = \frac{E}{R_2}.$$

The battery supplies the total current I; so,

$$I = I_1 + I_2.$$

Substituting for I_1 and I_2;

$$I = \frac{E}{R_1} + \frac{E}{R_2},$$

and

$$I = E\left(\frac{1}{R_1} + \frac{1}{R_2}\right) = E\left(\frac{R_2 + R_1}{R_1 R_2}\right),$$

or

$$E = I\left(\frac{R_1 R_2}{R_1 + R_2}\right).$$

Therefore,

$$Re = \frac{R_1 R_2}{R_1 + R_2}.$$

If

$$R_1 = R_2 = 100\ \Omega$$

and

$$E = 12\ \text{V}.$$

Then

$$I_1 = I_2 = \frac{12\ \text{V}}{100\ \Omega} = 0.12\ \text{A}$$

and

$$P_1 = P_2 = 0.12\ \text{A} \times 12\ \text{V} = 1.44\ \text{W}.$$

11(b). When the control switch is operated the coil current builds up exponentially with a time constant L/R, in this case,

$$\frac{60 \times 10^{-3}\ \text{H}}{100\ \Omega} = 0.6\ \text{ms}.$$

The current starts at zero, and builds up to a steady state value of

$$I = \frac{V}{R} = \frac{12\ \text{V}}{100\ \Omega} = 0.12\ \text{A}.$$

A current of 0.114 A is

$$\frac{0.114}{0.12} = 95\%$$

of the steady state value. From Chapter 3 and Figure 20 we know that 95 percent of the final value of an exponential rise curve is reached in three time constants. The coil currently builds up in

$$3 \times 0.6 \quad \text{ms} = 1.8 \text{ ms},$$

to a value of 0.114 A and operates the relay switch.

12. The electrical circuit shown in Figure 76 is a series A.C. circuit; a voltage rise, V_{in}, is opposed by the voltage drops of the resistor and capacitor. If we designate Vr as the voltage drop across the resistor, and Vc as the voltage drop across the capacitor, then Kirchoff's law states that

$$V_{in} = Vr + Vc.$$

Since this is a series circuit, a current I will flow through both R and C, and Ohm's law applied to the A.C. circuit yields

$$Vr = IR, \text{ and } Vc = IXc.$$

Now IR is in phase with V_{in}, but IXc lags V_{in} by 90° as shown in Figure 104. The impedance Z of R and C in series will be the vector addition of Xc and R which are at right angles; that is,

$$Z = \sqrt{R^2 + Xc^2}$$

Kirchoff's law may be restated as

$$V_{in} = IZ = I\sqrt{R^2 + Xc^2}.$$

We also know that $V_{out} = IXc$. The condition that $V_{out} = V_{in}/2$ may be stated as

$$IXc = I\sqrt{R^2 + Xc^2} \ / \ 2$$

or

$$Xc = \sqrt{R^2 + Xc^2} \ / \ 2$$

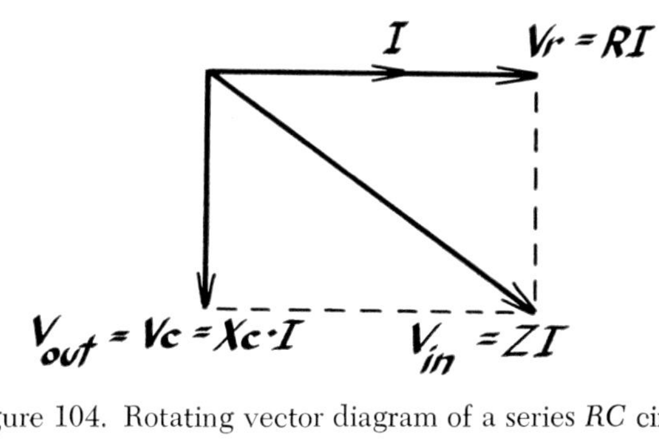

Figure 104. Rotating vector diagram of a series *RC* circuit.

Simplifying,

$$2Xc = \sqrt{R^2 + Xc^2},$$

square both sides,

$$4Xc^2 = R^2 + Xc^2,$$

$$3Xc^2 = R^2,$$

take the root of both sides,

$$\sqrt{3}\, Xc = R,$$

but,

$$Xc = 1/2\pi fC,$$

therefore,

$$\sqrt{3} = 2\pi RfC,$$

and

$$f = \sqrt{3}/2\pi RC.$$

Substituting the values of R and C

$$f = \sqrt{3}/2\pi \cdot 10^4 \cdot 10^{-6},$$

$$f = 27.5 \text{ Hz}.$$

We conclude that the transmission of rapid pressure fluctuations in a blood pressure cannula is impaired by the presence of air bubbles.

13. The electromyogram has a signal frequency range of 10 to 5 kHz according to Table XVII. Both the amplifier and recorder must have bandwidths in excess of this requirement. The recorder must be either an oscilloscope and camera or a galvanometer recorder.

The signal to be amplified is a bioelectric potential resulting from quite small movements of charge. The input impedance of the amplifier must therefore be large. It is most likely that the E.M.G. will be recorded in an electrically noisy environment so in order to minimize A.C. pickup, a differential amplifier should be chosen.

INDEX

O

P

Q

R

S

W

X